Diagnostic Testing

Guest Editor

STEPHEN D. KRAU, PhD, RN, CNE, CT

CRITICAL CARE NURSING CLINICS OF NORTH AMERICA

www.ccnursing.theclinics.com

Consulting Editor
JANET FOSTER, PhD, RN, CNS

March 2010 • Volume 22 • Number 1

SAUNDERS an imprint of ELSEVIER, Inc.

W.B. SAUNDERS COMPANY
A Division of Elsevier Inc.

Elsevier Inc., 1600 John F. Kennedy Blvd., Suite 1800, Philadelphia, PA 19103-2899

http://www.theclinics.com

CRITICAL CARE NURSING CLINICS OF NORTH AMERICA Volume 22, Number 1
March 2010 ISSN 0899-5885, ISBN-13: 978-1-4377-1808-9

Editor: Katie Hartner
Developmental Editor: Donald Mumford

Critical Care Nursing Clinics of North America (ISSN 0899-5885) is published quarterly by Elsevier Inc., 360 Park Avenue South, New York, NY 10010-1710. Months of issue are March, June, September, and December. Business and Editorial Offices: 1600 John F. Kennedy Blvd., Suite 1800, Philadelphia, PA 19103-2899. Periodicals postage paid at New York, NY and additional mailing offices. Subscription prices are $130.00 per year for US individuals, $256.00 per year for US institutions, $68.00 per year for US students and residents, $167.00 per year for Canadian individuals, $321.00 per year for Canadian institutions, $191.00 per year for international individuals, $321.00 per year for international institutions and $99.00 per year for Canadian and foreign students/residents. To receive student/resident rate, orders must be accompanied by name of affiliated institution, data of term, and the *signature* of program/residency coordinator on institution letterhead. Orders will be billed at individual rate until proof of status is received. Foreign air speed delivery is included in all *Clinics* subscription prices. All prices are subject to change without notice. **POSTMASTER:** Send address changes to *Critical Care Nursing Clinics of North America*, Elsevier Health Sciences Division, Subscription Customer Service, 3251 Riverport Lane, Maryland Heights, MO 63043. **Customer Service: 1-800-654-2452 (US and Canada); 314-447-8871 (outside US and Canada). Fax: 314-447-8029. E-mail: JournalsCustomerService-usa@elsevier.com (for print support) and JournalsOnlineSupport-usa@elsevier.com (for online support).**

Reprints. For copies of 100 or more of articles in this publication, please contact the Commercial Reprints Department, Elsevier Inc., 360 Park Avenue South, New York, New York, 10010-1710; Tel.: (212) 633-3813, Fax: (212) 462-1935, and E-mail: reprints@elsevier.com.

Critical Care Nursing Clinics of North America is covered in *MEDLINE/PubMed (Index Medicus)*, *International Nursing Index, Nursing Citation Index, Cumulative Index to Nursing and Allied Health Literature,* and *RNdex Top 100.*

Printed in the United States of America.

Contributors

CONSULTING EDITOR

JANET FOSTER, PhD, RN, CNS
Associate Professor, College of Nursing, Texas Women's University, Houston, Texas

GUEST EDITOR

STEPHEN D. KRAU, PhD, RN, CNE, CT
Associate Professor of Nursing, School of Nursing, Vanderbilt University Medical Center, Nashville, Tennessee

AUTHORS

CATHY A. COOPER, EdD, MSN, RN, CNE
Associate Professor, School of Nursing, Middle Tennessee State University, Murfreesboro, Tennessee

FRANCISCA CISNEROS FARRAR, EdD, MSN
Professor of Nursing, Austin Peay State University; Director of Nursing, School of Nursing, Austin Peay State University, Clarksville, Tennessee

DEBORAH ELLISON, MSN
Assistant Professor of Adult Health Nursing, School of Nursing, Austin Peay State University, Clarksville, Tennessee

AMY S. HAMLIN, MSN, RN
School of Nursing, Austin Peay State University, Clarksville, Tennessee

MARY ANN JESSEE, MSN, RN
Instructor of Nursing, Vanderbilt University School of Nursing, Nashville, Tennessee

STEPHEN D. KRAU, PhD, RN, CNE, CT
Associate Professor of Nursing, School of Nursing, Vanderbilt University Medical Center, Nashville, Tennessee

LEIGH ANN McINNIS, PhD, RN, FNP-BC
Associate Professor of Nursing and Associate Director Online Programs, Middle Tennessee State University, School of Nursing, Murfreesboro, Tennessee

GRACE MOODT, MSN
Assistant Professor of Adult Health Nursing, School of Nursing, Austin Peay State University, Clarksville, Tennessee

PATTY ORR, EdD
Chair of Excellence for the School of Nursing, Assistant Professor of Nursing, Austin Peay State University, Clarksville, Tennessee

LYNN PARSONS, DSN, RN, NE-BC
Professor and Director, Middle Tennessee State University, School of Nursing, Murfreesboro, Tennessee

MARCIA PUGH, MSN, MBA, HCM
Director, Grants, Research and Outreach of West AL Division, Tombigbee Healthcare Authority, Demopolis, Alabama

MARIA A. REVELL, DSN, RN, COI
Professor, School of Nursing, Middle Tennessee State University, Murfreesboro, Tennessee

TAMARA M. ROBERTSON, MSN, APN, FNP-BC, CUNP
School of Nursing, Austin Peay State University, Clarksville, Tennessee

SANDRA R. SCHOLTEN, MSN, FNP-BC
Lecturer, Instructor of Nursing, Vanderbilt School of Nursing, Nashville, Tennessee

TASHA L. SMITH, BS
Clinical Trial Leader, Cardiac Management, Medtronic, Coral Sea North East, Mounds View, Minnesota

MELAN SMITH-FRANCIS, MSN
Assistant Professor of Maternal Child Nursing, School of Nursing, Austin Peay State University, Clarksville, Tennessee

DIXIE L. TAYLOR, BSN, RN
Assistant Manager, Department of Medical Intensive Care, Vanderbilt University Medical Center, Nashville, Tennessee

MICHELLE L. WILLIAMS, MSN
Assistant Professor of Adult Health Nursing, School of Nursing, Austin Peay State University, Clarksville, Tennessee

XIAOHUA WU, MSN, FNP-BC
Lecturer, Vanderbilt University School of Nursing; Associate Professor, Vanderbilt University School of Nursing; Vanderbilt University Kidney Transplant Center, Nashville, Tennessee

Contents

A cornerstone in the quest for evidence is the use of diagnostic tests to determine the underlying issue for any symptoms seen in a patient. Clearly, diagnosis is not the final outcome in any patient scenario, but rather the beginning. The purpose of diagnostic testing is to provide evidence that will guide the health care provider in decision-making that will lead to achieving positive patient outcomes. This article provides a process by which a diagnostic test can be evaluated within the parameters of a patient condition. Through a thorough understanding of the test, the critical care nurse can be more effective in educating the patient, preparing the patient, and anticipating post-procedure nursing interventions for the patient undergoing diagnostic testing.

This article overviews electrodiagnostic tests that provide evidence-based data in the treatment and management of abnormalities in nerves and muscles. There is a focused review on cardiac tests, nerve-conduction tests, low-back pain tests, seizure and epilepsy tests, and obstructive sleep apnea electrodiagnostic tests. Case reports demonstrate how these electrophysiologic tests can provide specific data about the location and underlying causative factors of abnormalities in the nerves and muscles that routine diagnostic tests cannot differentiate.

As an invasive procedure, endoscopic studies require patient care and considerations that are very similar to minor surgical procedures. There are some general guidelines that are applicable to all endoscopic procedures, and there are special considerations that are dictated by the specific endoscopic procedure. It is important for the critical care nurse to understand the procedures because the differences and similarities of each procedure guide nursing actions to effect the best patient outcomes.

Although bronchoscopies have been performed for over a century and are relatively safe when practice guidelines are followed, they are invasive and a real source of anxiety and fear for the patient. The role of the critical care

nurse is essential to a successful outcome. This article provides an overview of the main diagnostic and therapeutic indications, contraindications,
and possible complications. Also discussed are patient education; patient
and staff safety; and considerations before, during, and after the
procedure.

Critical care patients present with or develop conditions that require imaging with a variety of radiographic methods. Technological advances such
as the introduction of digital imaging instead of screen-film radiography
have improved image resolution, readability, management, and portability
of results while maintaining confidentiality of patient information. Radiographic imaging in the critical care unit is an integral part of patient management. It is imperative that the critical care nurse be cognizant of
radiographic studies and thus be able to collaborate with all health care
providers in the administration of quality patient care.

In critical care, nurses are expected to react quickly to urgent and emergent situations. It is imperative that nurses have the ability to recognize
signs and symptoms in patients that require diagnostic intervention. This
article begins with a brief description of angiography and its role in the critical care environment. This is followed by a description and comparison of
several modalities used to evaluate the cerebral and carotid vessels. A related case study, from a patient's perspective, provides the context for this
discussion.

The field of nuclear cardiology has grown significantly over the past decade.
This is a reflection of the value seen by providers in these safe and effective
procedures. Nuclear scan studies are noninvasive and versatile in their usefulness. These studies assist in determining the likelihood of future cardiac
events, guide approaches to revascularization, and assist in evaluation of
the adequacy of revascularization procedures. Critical thinking and decision-making abilities are two key requirements for nurses in the critical
care environment. Knowledge and understanding of the nuclear scan studies indicated for patients help nurses advocate for those in their care.

Skin testing is a common procedure in any clinical setting. Critical care
nurses will encounter skin testing in the inpatient and outpatient settings

primarily to test for patient allergies to environmental factors, or allergies to certain medications. As there is a great deal of controversy about standard practices surrounding the different tests, information about various allergy tests and testing protocols is vital. Quality assurance standards should be met to ensure adequacy of the skin testing technique. Persons performing skin tests should undergo evaluation of their technique. To improve the predictive values of skin testing, and to ameliorate the incidence or severity of adverse affects, it is important for the critical care nurse to understand the dynamics of the test and the possible risks, along with variables that can confound the results. By doing this, nurses will improve not only patient outcomes related to the testing itself but also the value and reliability of the most effective diagnostic tool available for allergic disease.

This article focuses on the clinical use of ultrasound with the obstetric, gynecologic, and trauma patient by reviewing recent case studies of the use of ultrasound for diagnostic purposes. The article also summarizes the American Institute of Ultrasound in Medicine (AIUM) guidelines for use in several types of patients. The AIUM is a multidisciplinary association whose purpose is to "advance the art and science of ultrasound in medicine and research through educational, scientific, literary, and professional activities." The organization provides guidelines in conjunction with many professional organizations, such as the American College of Cardiology and the American College of Obstetrics and Gynecology. AIUM also serves as an accrediting body for ultrasound practices.

Critical care nurses have a vital role in caring for patients undergoing centesis studies. Any centesis procedure involves puncturing a body cavity, joint, organ, or space with a hollow needle to withdraw fluid. All centesis studies are invasive procedures, typically performed for either therapeutic or diagnostic purposes. Because there are a variety of centesis procedures that the critical care nurse might encounter, the following centesis procedures are discussed in depth: amniocentesis, arthrocentesis, lumbar puncture, paracentesis, pericardiocentesis, and thoracentesis. By becoming more familiar with each of these procedures, the critical care nurse gains confidence in caring for clients when these procedures are indicated.

Voiding dysfunction has profound physical, emotional, and financial ramifications for patients and health care practitioners from all fields. The improvement of diagnostic testing in the area of voiding dysfunction, throughout decades, has resulted in improved patient outcomes. The components of urodynamic studies can allow practitioners an objective measurement to assist in making a correct diagnosis, hence appropriate interventions. An urodynamic study decreases the risk of a patient undergoing unnecessary surgical procedures. Urodynamics is an invasive procedure, though with the maintenance of sterile technique and patient education it is generally well tolerated with few adverse effects.

Xiaohua Wu

There is much value in using urine as a diagnostic aid in the critical care setting. As a noninvasive source of data, urine reveals a wealth of information about the body's biochemical status. It is important for critical care nurses to understand the processes that occur in the renal system and to comprehend the depth of information that can be obtained through an analysis of urine. This discussion provides an overview of common urine tests and provides information for nurses about urine collection methods. The discussion will help the critical care nurse describe various urine test procedures, common urine collection methods, nursing interventions, and patient education important to each study.

Mary Ann Jessee

Much information can be obtained about a patient's gastrointestinal and overall nutritional status through stool samples. Important infectious processes and neoplastic processes are initially identified through diagnostic tests and screening of stool samples. Although in some arenas they are a source of embarrassment and distaste, the value of correctly obtained samples is unquestionable. Patient collaboration with a critical care nurse is integral to obtaining stool samples.

Preface

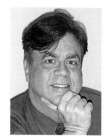

Stephen D. Krau, PhD, RN, CNE, CT
Guest Editor

Diagnostic tests in the broadest sense consist of any method of gathering information that may change or confirm a clinician's view about the likelihood that a patient has a particular condition. The tests are not the ends in themselves, but do provide genuine evidence that should lead to clinical decisions that improve patient outcomes. Diagnostic tests are the cornerstone of evidence-based practice. As such, these tests should be considered with the same rigor as therapeutic interventions. The critical care nurse has a pivotal role in diagnostic testing, be it something simple, like a urine specimen collection, or something more technologically complex, such as a bronchoscope or imaging study. Appropriate patient preparation and understanding, and proper testing procedures are imperative for reliable testing results and patient safety. A thorough plan of care for a patient undergoing any sort of diagnostic test must include education about the procedure, preparation for the test, information about what the patient can anticipate during the test, information about postprocedure expectations, and potential results. The quality of patient education is contingent upon the nurse's understanding of the procedure, rapport with the patient, and ability to discern and address patient concerns and questions regarding the test and testing procedure.

This issue of *Critical Care Nursing Clinics of North America* is devoted to enhancing the understanding of selected diagnostic tests that many nurses encounter and that are often seen in critical care settings. Discussions are not limited to the diagnostic and sometimes therapeutic capabilities of the tests, but extend to the nursing responsibilities related to correct management of the tests, patient education before and after the tests, and an overview about the purpose of the tests, as well as the specificity and sensitivity of the tests. The purpose of each article is to inform the nurse thoroughly about the test so that the patient for whom the nurse is caring can benefit.

Issues related to diagnostic testing are multifold. Currently, there is concern that diagnostic tests need only prove they measure a given analyte, and that the test may or may not be of use in managing patient outcomes. As such, there are constituents who believe that diagnostic testing should have the same model for "license" in clinical use as medications. In fact, they maintain that a pharmaceutical model should be used to determine a clinical test for use.[1] Although no health care agencies in the United States regulate the use or appropriateness of diagnostic testing, appropriate

doi:10.1016/j.ccell.2009.10.014

ccnursing.theclinics.com

and judicious diagnostic testing is imperative in today's milieu with the emphasis on costs and cost containment. Additionally, extraneous testing may reveal information not warranted in the patient situation, information that has the potential to result in negative consequences emotionally and physically. For these reasons, it is important that diagnostic testing be selected appropriately, be executed appropriately, and be evaluated properly.

It falls within the scope of a nurse's responsibility to ensure the patient is properly prepared for the test. This means that the patient not only be physically prepared, but also be informed about the test so he or she can participate in the decision to have the test. The patient should know the risks involved in testing, and should understand the purpose of the test. This falls within the realm of ethical and legal processes with regard to informed consent. Many issues surround informed consent, but only through the ability to answer patient questions and explain procedures to patients can nurses effect patient understanding. Additionally, if patients have knowledge of the procedure and what is expected, they are more likely to contribute to the process as appropriate. One cannot deny the value of a noncatheterized patient understanding and cooperating with something even as simple as a 24-hour urine collection. Breaches in specimen collection for a 24-hour urine collection have resulted in extended hospital stays, delayed diagnosis, and increased stress to the patient. On the other end of the spectrum, a patient who does not understand the importance of having nothing by mouth before a bronchoscope, might eat or drink before the procedure. If this is unknown to the nurse, there is a certain safety risk of patient aspiration. In cases where this becomes known and the procedure is postponed, the result is a delay in patient diagnosis, the potential for an extended hospital stay, and increased patient and staff stress. Beyond this, a cancellation can affect the system flow of patients awaiting the same procedure. Both testing scenarios effect costs and can be averted by clear instruction and certain confirmation of patient understanding.

The critical care nurse needs to know the testing process and procedure to be sure that a patient does not have a condition or has not engaged in an activity that makes the test invalid or effects patient safety. Factors relevant to testing can be simple, such as patient allergies or when the patient last ate or drank, or subtle, such as the patient's anticoagulant regimen, religious or cultural considerations, or insidious change in status discerned only by the nurse who is caring for the patient.

This issue covers many common diagnostic tests and will serve as both a review for some nurses and as new information for others. It is not meant to be a handbook or to replace laboratory manuals, but rather as a source of comprehensive information about a myriad of diagnostic tests that provide foundational evidence. It is the goal of this issue to provide or enhance foundational knowledge of diagnostic testing that will be used to effect quality nursing care and positive patient outcomes.

Stephen D. Krau, PhD, RN, CNE, CT
School of Nursing
Vanderbilt University Medical Center
314 Godchaux Hall
461 21st Avenue
South Nashville, TN 37240, USA

E-mail address:
steve.krau@vanderbilt.edu

REFERENCE

1. Gluud C, Gluud LL. Evidence based diagnostics. BMJ 2005;330:724–6.

Diagnostic Testing: The Search for Real Evidence

Stephen D. Krau, PhD, RN, CNE, CT

KEYWORDS

• Diagnostic tests • Sensitivity • Specificity • Evidence-based

With the current emphasis on evidence in evidence-based practice, the value of the evidence is mostly perceived as most information that is supportive of specific medications and that which confirms the value and validity of medical and nursing interventions. In reality, the pursuit for sound evidence occurs the moment the patient comes in contact with the health care system, and continues throughout diagnosis and treatment. A cornerstone in the quest for evidence is the use of diagnostic tests to determine the underlying issue for any symptoms seen in a patient. Clearly, diagnosis is not the final outcome in any patient scenario, but rather the beginning. The purpose of diagnostic testing is to guide the health care provider in decision-making that will lead to achieving positive patient outcomes. Because they are fundamental to any patient care scenario, diagnostic tests warrant the same scrutiny and appraisal used to judge the value any therapeutic intervention. Currently, there is no international consensus on the methods by which diagnostic tests should be evaluated. Previous recommendations maintain that diagnostic tests should match the type of diagnostic question.[1,2] Whereas this is essential, this is not enough in the current health care milieu where health care costs are a major consideration.

Although the name diagnostic test implies diagnosis only, the true value of any test lies in its ability to not only diagnose but also its ability to guide the health care provider toward prognostic and therapeutic decisions. To facilitate this purpose, it is crucial that all health care providers understand the basics of diagnostic testing, regardless of the test, and that nurses comprehend their responsibilities in situations that require diagnostic testing. In the critical care setting, where patients are continually assessed and participate in diagnostic testing, this is particularly central because the reliability and validity of the test is contingent on several factors discussed in this article.

Vanderbilt University Medical Center, 314 Godchaux Hall, 461 21st Avenue South, Nashville, TN 37240, USA

E-mail address: steve.krau@vanderbilt.edu

Crit Care Nurs Clin N Am 22 (2010) 1–6

doi:10.1016/j.ccell.2009.10.005

ccnursing.theclinics.com

0899-5885/10/$ – see front matter © 2010 Elsevier Inc. All rights reserved.

THE SCIENTIFIC BASE FOR DIAGNOSTIC ACCURACY

The viability of a diagnostic test lies in its ability to impact clinical management, patient outcome, and overall well-being of the patient. Tests that do not meet these requirements become obsolete quickly. An essential quality of any diagnostic test involves the accuracy of the test. Unlike medications that are subject to great scrutiny and review, diagnostic tests are not. Among the measures of accuracy for diagnostic tests are sensitivity and specificity. Sensitivity is the probability that there will be a positive test result in a target population, and specificity is the probability of a negative test result in the absence of a target condition.[3]

The scientific base for the accuracy of diagnostic tests has grown tremendously over the last several years with special attention given to the impact of bias and variation on the specific test.[4–6] There has been a great deal of discussion about the design of diagnostic accuracy studies.[7–11] Variation and bias in studies of diagnostic accuracy and diagnostic testing accuracy continue to be topics of much discussion.[12] Owing to inconclusive rigor in the studies used to appraise the value of tests, along with the poor reporting and inappropriate dissemination, the Standards for Reporting of Diagnostic Accuracy initiative,[13] and the Grading of Recommendations Assessment, Development and Evaluation system[14] have emerged. A rigorous evaluation of diagnostic tests, and ongoing evaluation of these tests for subgroups, could lead to lower health care costs and better clinical consequences.

The evaluation of the accuracy of a test is only one aspect of its potential for clinical value. When considering treatment interventions in the health care setting, the value of the intervention is only supported if the intervention is considered to be of benefit to the patient. As a guide for the clinician, even the most accurate diagnostic test can be clinically useless if it does not yield important information or if the test does more harm than good. The accuracy of any test is only one aspect of its value in clinical practice.

EVALUATING THE APPROPRIATENESS OF A DIAGNOSTIC TEST IN THE CRITICAL CARE SETTING

Fundamental to diagnostic testing is the evaluation of the criteria that exists to perform the test. This information comes from the patient's complaints or symptoms. This information is foundational to the type of test that should be considered. The appropriate test is contingent on the information that is sought in each clinical situation. This, in itself, seems basic and logical, but the choice of test or tests is contingent on many factors. As there is no standard or regulatory body that determines the value of diagnostic tests in variant circumstances, it is essential that the clinician evaluate the information that is to be obtained from a specific test. The clinical value of the information obtained from a test can only be as valuable as the test itself and the clear standards by which a test is performed or executed. The patient preparation for testing, the procedures and protocols for the test, and the follow-up care of the patient undergoing a diagnostic test are important facets of testing for the critical care nurse.

There are many methods and models for evaluating the value of a diagnostic test itself. The method proposed by Van den Bruel and colleagues[4] is a stepwise method where one step leads to the next and, to progress, there must be evidence to support moving to the next step. Although the scheme is designed to evaluate a new test, it parallels considerations for the implementation of the test in a patient care scenario. In other words, the same criteria for assessing the value of a new test, is parallel to the criteria for introducing a test into the patient scenario. Although the test under consideration might not be considered a new test, it is new to the patient scenario as a potential diagnostic tool.

Technical Accuracy

As described by Van den Bruel and colleagues,[4] this step involves understanding the ability of the test to provide useful information under laboratory conditions or under the perfect scenario. Considerations include the ability of the test to detect a specific quantity of what is expected to be measured and the specificity of the test to indicate components other than the specified target that may cause false results. The critical care nurse should know about the tests and the proper procedure for collecting, assisting, or performing the tests. Variations in these can corrupt the findings of the test and make the findings inaccurate.

As with quality research, another component of the technical accuracy of the test lies in the reproducibility of the test. This is the degree to which the test will obtain the same results, providing there is no change in the patient or testing procedure, in repeated cases or observations. Reproducibility with any tests is also influenced by systematic and random error. There is a variety of resources available to nurses to determine the technical accuracy of any test. Some of these resources can be found in the literature, among regulatory agencies, and authoritative resources.

Placement of the Test in the Clinical Pathway

In the scheme proposed by Van de Bruel and colleagues,[4] this step refers to the determination of the needed characteristics of the new test, the information already present, and the information still needed. The parallel to clinical practice is clear because this involves the overall goal of the test for the patient: the indications for the new test, the information that indicates the test should be performed, and a clear understanding of what information is to be obtained from the test result and how this will be used. The parallel scheme indicates that a new test will either replace an existing test in the clinical pathway, be used before the pathway as triage, or be used after the pathway as an add-on.[4,8]

In the patient care setting, the parallel demonstrates that a new test that has been ordered or considered has value in the discovery of evidence or providing new information to support the clinical pathway. The test may be useful to triage a group of patients or help set priorities for interventions for an individual patient. A newly ordered test may be a measure to exclude competing ideas or notions related to the diagnosis, go beyond the common reference standard, and be warranted owing to subgroup variations among patients. The add-on test might be one that is more expensive, and more invasive than earlier tests but considered because of the value of the information that will be provided.

Diagnostic Accuracy

In the scheme proposed by Van de Bruel and colleagues,[4] diagnostic accuracy refers to the test's ability to detect or exclude a disease or target condition in patients. At this step, the test is compared with a reference standard or with a set of patients for whom the test indicates or completely rules out a certain disease or condition. In this scheme, a new test is assessed primarily as a replacement of an existing test, to triage patients before the existing pathway, or as an add-on test. As an add-on test, the characteristics that are desired depend on the goal of the test. Hopefully, the add-on test will increase sensitivity by decreasing the number of patients testing falsely negative and increase specificity by decreasing the number of patients who test falsely positive.[4]

In the clinical setting, this step encompasses the notion that diagnostic accuracy is the ability of the test to correctly detect or exclude a target condition or disease in patients.[4] It is helpful to consider this in relation to the patient's clinical pathway.

The concepts of sensitivity and specificity are important to this step. If a new test is introduced, the health care provider should consider all options when making the decision as to the particulars of the test. For example, ordering a urine culture and sensitivity along with a urinalysis indicates the need for more specific information than can be obtained by an urinalysis alone.

With regard to the clinical pathway of the patient, if a new test is to replace an existing test, a review of all similar tests is warranted. Comparisons of all tests related to the symptom or issue should be considered. This increases the value of the test and could ameliorate issues related to excessive testing. Diagnostic accuracy also has implications for diagnosticians because this may result in withholding unneeded treatment.

With regard to triage, the test can be used to evaluate and prioritize among a group of patients or to set priorities within one case. In cases of comorbidities, it can be used to determine which condition, disease, or process takes priority. The test itself does not make that determination, but the test yields information to the clinician that should be used to make decisions.

Adding a test to a patient scenario warrants clear justification. If there is a need to increase the sensitivity and specificity in the patient case for better treatment, a test that is intended as an add-on might be considered. Issues related to add-on tests in these ambiguous situations include the potential for more invasiveness and increase in costs. However, if the information yields direction toward a more effective and targeted treatment, then performing the test is weighed against these issues.

Impact on Patient Outcome

The main goal of the diagnostic test is to contribute information that will improve patient outcome. The impact on the outcome should be considered against the risks of the test, including the potential for pain, risk, expected harm, or cost of the test. The benefits against which the risks are measured include improved life expectancy, quality of life, and avoidance of additional tests or procedures. In some cases, the only benefit may be to give the patient a clear diagnosis of the situation.[4] The critical care nurse who is caring for a patient undergoing a diagnostic test, should have a clear understanding of the purpose of the test, along with the risks and benefits to the patient.

Cost-effectiveness

The fifth step in evaluating the usefulness of a diagnostic test, centers on the cost-effectiveness. This is an interesting placement for this step because cost is considered a major problem facing health care in many countries. Global inflation, increased number of elderly, new technology, and marketing are only some of the variables that affect cost related to diagnostic testing. The impact of diagnostic testing, and the subsequent costs, goes far beyond individual patient risks and benefits.[4] Tests should be considered with regard to specialized education and training needed by staff for the specific tests, the availability of the tests to society as whole, and the affordability to persons regardless of different financial means and resources. A goal within this step is avoiding overtesting, and undertesting. Testing done solely for the sake of professional liability concerns should be avoided.[15] Some data suggests that up to 50% of the analyses performed daily in clinical laboratories may be inappropriate.[16]

THE PROCESS

Although intended to provide research guidance for the development and the evaluation of new and proven diagnostic tests, the scheme provided by Van de Bruel and colleagues[4] provides guidance to the clinical decision-making about the tests that are considered in each patient scenario. As a vital member of the health care team, it is imperative that the critical care nurse understands the process and can articulate the purpose, patient expectations, and potential outcomes as they relate to caring for the critical care patient. With the current effect of costs on health care, the cost-effectiveness step may take priority over the other steps. In cases where patients are uninsured or underinsured, there may be less possibility that a test is offered. This is a reality in the current health care environment.

PATIENT CONSENT FOR TESTING

With regard to diagnostic testing and health care, the quality of care improves when there is clear communication and mutual understanding between the health care provider and the patient.[15] The relationship is mutual as the health care provider and the patient have the responsibility to work toward the same goal, to be open, and to be honest. In order for this to occur, there must be information from the health care provider that promotes a relationship of honesty and trust. Likewise, the patient is responsible for providing thorough and accurate information that may affect the judgment of the health care provider.[4] The critical care nurse who is caring for a patient undergoing a diagnostic test, should have a clear understanding of the purpose of the test, along with the risks and benefits to the patient.

Any test that is ordered should be directed to providing information about the patient, for the benefit of the patient.[15] There are circumstances in which third parties might request information obtained from diagnostic tests, including insurance companies, employers, or extended family members. In these cases, the test is performed within ethical guidelines when the patient or proxy understands the potential risks and benefits and gives consent.[15] Informed consent continues to be an ongoing issue, not only for diagnostic testing, but also in cases where there are strict guidelines for obtaining informed consent, such as clinical trials. The current methods for obtaining consent, defining consent, and measuring comprehension are inadequate.[17]

SUMMARY

This clinical decision-making process parallels the steps in assessing the use and value of a new diagnostic test. With no current regulatory constraints on diagnostic testing, whether a test is to be done is based on the clinical decision-maker and, pragmatically, the availability of the test or resources and cost of the test. Critical care nurses can use this process in understanding the test, how it fits into the patient's plan of care, and how the test is used to contribute to positive patient outcomes. The process helps inform the nurse who, in turn, should be teaching the patient, preparing the patient for the test, and anticipating posttesting procedure responsibilities.

REFERENCES

1. Sackett D, Haynes RB. The architecture of diagnostic research. BMJ 2002;324: 539–41.
2. Gluud C, Gluud LL. Evidence based diagnostics. BMJ 2005;330:724–6.
3. Biesheuval C, Irwig L, Bossuyt P. Observed differences in diagnostic test accuracy between patient subgroups: is it real or due to reference standard misclassification. Clin Chem 2007;53(10):1725–9.

4. Van den Bruel A, Cleempt I, Aertgeerts B, et al. The evaluation of diagnostic tests: evidence on technical and diagnostic accuracy, impact on patient outcome and cost-effectiveness is needed. J Clin Epidemiol 2007;60:1116–22.
5. Lijmer JG, Mol BW, Heisterkamp S, et al. Empirical evidence of design-related bias in studies of diagnostic tests. JAMA 1999;282:1061–6.
6. Rutjes AW, Reitsma JB, Di Nisio M, et al. Evidence of bias and variation in diagnostic accuracy studies. CMAJ 2006;174:469–76.
7. Rutjes AW, Reitsma JB, Vandenbroucke JP, et al. Case-control and two-gate designs in diagnostic accuracy studies. Clin Chem 2005;51:1335–41.
8. Bossuyt PM, Irwig L, Craig J, et al. Comparative accuracy: assessing new tests against existing diagnostic pathways. BMJ 2006;332:1089–92.
9. Irwig LM, Bossuyt PM, Glasziou PP, et al. Designing studies to ensure that estimates of test accuracy will travel. In: Knottnerus JA, editor. The evidence base of clinical diagnosis. Boston: BMJ Books; 2002. p. 95–116.
10. Moons KG, Biesheuvel CJ, Grobbee DE. Test research versus diagnostic research. Clin Chem 2004;50:473–6.
11. Knottnerus JA, Muris JW. Assessment of the accuracy of diagnostic tests: the cross-sectional study. J Clin Epidemiol 2003;56:1118–28.
12. Whiting P, Rutjes A, Johannes B, et al. Sources of variation and bias in studies of diagnostic accuracy: a systematic review. Ann Intern Med 2004;140:189–202.
13. Bossuyt PM, Reitsma JB, Bruns DE, et al. Towards complete and accurate reporting of studies of diagnostic accuracy: the STARD initiative. BMJ 2003;326:41–4.
14. Schünemann A, Oxman A, Brozek J, et al. Grading quality of evidence and strength of recommendations for diagnostic tests and strategies. BMJ 2008;336:1106–10.
15. American College of Obstetricians and Gynecologists. Patient testing: ethical issues in selection and counseling. Obstet Gynecol 2007;109(4):1021–3.
16. Plebani M, Ceriotti F, Messeri G, et al. Laboratory network of excellence: enhancing patient safety and service effectiveness. Clin Chem Lab Med 2006;44:150–60.
17. Cohn E, Larson E. Improving participant comprehension in the informed consent process. J Nurs Scholarsh 2007;39(3):273–80.

Electrodiagnostic Studies

Deborah Ellison, MSN, Michelle L. Williams, MSN*,
Grace Moodt, MSN, Francisca Cisneros Farrar, EdD, MSN

KEYWORDS

- Electrophysiology • Electrodiagnostic • Studies
- Nerves • Muscles

OVERVIEW OF ELECTRODIAGNOSTIC TESTS

Electrophysiology is the study of the electrical properties of biologic cells and tissues. It involves the measurement of voltage change or electric current on a wide variety of scales from single ion channel proteins to neurons firing in whole organs, such as the heart measuring the integrity of the conduction system. Electrodiagnostic tests are electrophysiologic studies of the electrical activity and conduction system of nerves and muscles at rest and during activity. These diagnostic tests provide significant evidence- based data for best-practice interventions in the treatment and management of abnormalities in nerves and muscles. Electrodiagnostic tests help provide specific data about the location and underlying causative factors of these abnormalities that routine diagnostic tests cannot differentiate.

There are few complications in electrodiagnostic tests. Noninvasive surface electrodes have rare complications. Patients are instructed not to wear lotion for 24 hours before the test. A complication might be an irritation or allergy to the adhesive of the electrode. Invasive complications are usually limited to the invasive procedure itself, such as insertion site infection and bleeding. A consent form is signed by patients after instruction is given about the procedure, complications, and follow-up care. The electrophysiology function of the target system area is usually produced in a graph format that requires a specialist to interpret. Most tests are conducted in an electrophysiology lab and interpreted by a trained specialist or electrophysiology physician. A disadvantage of electrodiagnostic tests is faculty interpretations of data caused by artifacts and an untrained reader of the test. The following summarizes common tests[1] in this graph format:

1. Electroantennography for the olfactory receptors in arthropods
2. Electrocardiography for the heart
3. Electrocorticography for the cerebral cortex
4. Electroencephalography for the brain

School of Nursing, Austin Peay State University, P.O. Box 4658, Clarksville, TN 37044, USA
* Corresponding author.
E-mail address: williamsm@apsu.edu (M.L. Williams).

Crit Care Nurs Clin N Am 22 (2010) 7–18
doi:10.1016/j.ccell.2009.10.011
0899-5885/10/$ – see front matter © 2010 Published by Elsevier Inc.

ccnursing.theclinics.com

5. Electromyography for the muscles
6. Electro-oculography for the eyes
7. Polysomnography, the gold standard diagnostic test for obstructive sleep apnea
8. Electroretinography for the retina

CARDIAC ELECTRODIAGNOSTIC STUDIES

Electrocardiography (ECG) is a common noninvasive electrodiagnostic test that records the electrical activity of the heart over time using skin electrodes. The ECG measures the overall rhythm of the heart in different parts of the heart muscle. It is a powerful diagnostic tool to diagnose abnormal rhythms of the heart. In myocardial infarction, the ECG can identify damaged heart muscle, ischemia, injury, or infarct. It can also identify electrolyte and drug level abnormalities. A 12 lead ECG is usually preliminary to most tests performed. It is used as a baseline diagnostic tool for identification of rhythms, and is often used as a comparison of pretest and posttest changes. A disadvantage of an ECG is that it cannot measure the pumping ability of the heart, and faculty interpretations can be made because of artifacts and an untrained reader of the electrocardiograph.[2]

Invasive cardiac electrophysiology diagnostic tests are used for diagnosis and treatment of cardiac rhythm disorders. Invasive cardiac electrophysiology procedures involve the introduction of an electrode catheter percutaneously from a peripheral vein or artery into the cardiac chamber of sinuses. These electrode catheters evaluate the performance of programmed electrical stimulation of the heart.[3] These electrophysiologic studies are used for seven primary diagnostic reasons:

1. Accurate diagnosis and management of bradyarrhythmias and tachyarrhythmias
2. Diagnosis of unknown etiology for syncope episodes
3. Determination of the prognosis of the cardiac rhythm disorder
4. Identification of risk factors for sudden cardiac death
5. Evidence-based data generation for primary prevention interventions, such as permanent pacemaker or defibrillator implantation
6. Electrophysiology data for drug-management decisions regarding antiarrhythmic drug therapy
7. Electrophysiology feasibility data for nonpharmacologic management of cardiac rhythm disorders, such as ablation or antiarrhythmic surgery.[3]

Invasive cardiac electrophysiology studies are usually performed in an electrophysiology laboratory using intravenous conscious sedation. The lab staff usually consists of an electrophysiologist physician, circulator nurse, nurse anesthetist, and another physician or technician. One of the staff continuously monitors patients' heart rhythm, and is able to defibrillate using a biphasic external defibrillator if needed. Multipolar intracardiac electrode catheters are positioned in the heart using the Seldinger technique to place multiple venous accesses. The femoral vascular access is the most common approach. Typical placement positions for the multipolar intracardiac electrode catheters include the right atrium (evaluate sinoatrial node function and atrioventricular conduction), right ventricle (useful site for adding premature stimuli during programmed ventricular stimulation), tricuspid annulus (record potential from the bundle of His), and coronary sinus (evaluate left atrial activation).[3]

Baseline recordings are obtained during the electrophysiology testing. The baseline recordings include several surface electrocardiograms and several intracardiac electrograms that are recorded simultaneously including the atrium, bundle of His, and ventricle. The electrophysiology diagnostic test measures four basic intervals that reflect the integrity of the conduction system under resting conditions.[3] The following list overviews these baseline measurements:

- PA interval is measured from the onset of the earliest P wave to the onset of the atrial deflection on the bundle of His recording. The normal range is 20 to 60 milliseconds. Prolonged PA times suggest abnormal atrial conduction such as first degree atrioventricular block.[3]
- AH interval measures the atrioventricular (AV) nodal conduction and is measured from the earliest deflection of the atrial recording to the earliest onset of the His bundle deflection. The normal range is 50 to 120 milliseconds. A short AH interval suggests abnormal AV nodal conduction which includes causative factors such as increased sympathetic tone and enhanced AV nodal conduction related to pregnancy and steroid use. A long-AH interval suggests abnormal AV nodal conduction that includes causative factors, such as enhanced vagal tone; intrinsic disease; and negative dromotropic drugs, such as amiodarone, digoxin, beta blockers, and calcium channel blockers.[3]
- His bundle of electrograms duration measures conduction through the short length of compact His bundle. The normal range is 15 to 25 milliseconds. Short and long His-bundle intervals suggest abnormalities in the His bundle conduction.[3]
- HV interval measures the conduction time through the distal His- Purkinje tissue and is measured from the onset of the His-bundle deflection to the earliest ventricular activation. The normal range is 35 to 55 milliseconds. A short-HV interval suggests ventricular preexcitation, such as premature ventricular contraction or an accelerated idioventricular rhythm.[3]

After completion of the baseline recordings, pacing is performed with the intracardiac electrode catheters with programmed electrical stimulation to assess AV conduction and to induce supraventricular and ventricular arrhythmias. Premature beats can be introduced by burst pacing and programmed electrical stimulation at various fixed-cycle lengths to investigate the electrophysiology of the tachycardia.[3] Complications of invasive electrophysiology studies are rare. Serious complications are usually related to the catheterization process of veins and arteries with a complication rate of approximately 2%.[3] Complications associated with percutaneous catheterization include pain, adverse drug reaction, infection/sepsis at the catheterization site, excessive bleeding, hematoma formation, thrombophlebitis, pulmonary thromboembolism, arterial damage, aortic dissection, systemic thromboembolism, transient ischemic attack, and stroke.[2] Complications associated with intracardiac catheters and programmed cardiac stimulation include cardiac chamber perforation, coronary sinus perforation, cardiac tamponade, atrial fibrillation, ventricular tachycardia, ventricular fibrillation, myocardial infarction, and right or left bundle branch block.[3] The induction of serious ventricular tachyarrhythmias occurs frequently and can be promptly terminated by overdrive pacing or external countershock.[3] A coronary angiography or echocardiography are recommended before the electrophysiology study in patients at risk for complications, such as patients who have ischemia or heart failure.

Mapping and transcatheter radiofrequency ablation commonly follows invasive cardiac electrophysiology testing in an attempt to alleviate the arrhythmia.[3] Radio frequency catheter ablation is the method of interrupting supraventricular tachycardia. The objective is to interrupt the two competing electrical conduction pathways.[2] A radiofrequency ablation is used to treat atrial fibrillation. Radiofrequency ablation is done in a circular pattern around each pulmonary vein where the lines of conduction abnormality are the contributing factors to atrial fibrillation.[2]

The electrophysiologic procedure begins with a diagnostic electrophysiology study. A catheter with an electrode is positioned at the abnormal pathway then painless radio frequency energy similar to microwave heat is transmitted through the pathway.[2] This ablation process causes coagulation and necrosis in the conduction fibers without destroying the surrounding tissue, which stops the area from conducting the extra impulses, thereby, alleviating the tachycardia.[2] Complications associated with trans-catheter radiofrequency ablation include complete heart block; thromboembolism; vascular access problems, such as bleeding, infection, and vascular injury; cardiac trauma, such as myocardial perforation and tamponade; myocardial infarction; cardiac arrhythmias; pericarditis; pulmonary vein stenosis; phrenic nerve paralysis; radiation skin burns; and death.[3]

Cardiac mapping is when the temporal and spatial distributions of electrical poten-tials generated by the myocardium during normal or abnormal rhythms are identified.[4,5] Cardiac mapping can detect myocardial activation and measures repolarization. Elec-trophysiologic cardiac mapping, including electroanatomic mapping, and noncontrast endocardial mapping, have replaced intraoperative mapping.[4] Invasive cardiac elec-trophysiology mapping and ablation is an established clinical technique for the inves-tigation and treatment of cardiac rhythm disorders. Invasive cardiac electrophysiology studies are used to diagnose and treat tachyarrhythmias, such as atrial fibrillation, atrial flutter, supraventricular tachycardia, and ventricular tachycardia.[4]

CASE REPORT: TACHYARRHYTHMIAS

DW, a 54-year-old woman, was recently diagnosed with a myocardial infarction resul-tant from ventricular tachycardia and right-sided heart failure. An echocardiogram revealed an ejection fraction of 24% with global dyskinesia. She presented to the cardiologist for her 4-week follow-up appointment post-hospitalization. DW reported that she has gained approximately 12 pounds since her second week after discharge and has been extremely fatigued with notable shortness of breath with any activity. Upon assessment, vital signs were stable. DW was dyspneic with an oxygen satura-tion of 91%. Lung fields displayed bilateral crackles in the bases. Heart tones were audible but distant and muffled. Lower extremities were edematous with three-plus pitting edema bilaterally, ruddy in color and cool to touch. Cardiac monitor revealed a rate of 115 beats per minute and normal sinus rhythm with frequent short runs of supraventricular tachycardia. DW had no evidence of advanced coronary disease. Based upon her recent diagnoses and current assessment findings, DW's cardiologist referred her for electrophysiology studies to review her cardiac conduction pattern.

Electrophysiology had a primary role in the management of DW's ventricular tachy-cardia. Therapeutic programmed stimulation and burst pacing can induce her ventric-ular tachycardia to provide electrophysiologic data for management of her ventricular tachycardia. This individualized evidence-based data can confirm her diagnosis and prognosis by determining the mechanism of the arrhythmia, define the hemodynamic instability during her ventricular tachycardia, provide cardiac mapping for transcath-eter ablation, provide data for the feasibility of an implantable cardioverter defibrillator (ICD) therapy, and guide antiarrhythmic drug therapy.

Invasive cardiac electrophysiology studies are also used in the treatment of bra-dyarrhythmias to determine if a permanent pacemaker is needed. Temporary pace-makers are used as an emergency basis to treat symptomatic bradycardia or to override tachydysrhythmias. Bradycardia results from heart block associated with cardiac abnormalities, such as anterior myocardial infarction, and digoxin toxicity. If symptomatic bradycardia continues despite treatment and resolution of cause, a permanent pacemaker is usually indicated.[2] Implantable cardioverter-defibrillators are used with patients who have life-threatening ventricular dysrhythmias, such as drug-refractory sustained ventricular or ventricular fibrillation. They are also used with a left-ventricular ejection fraction of 30% or less.[2]

Electrodiagnostic impulse formation and conduction intervals provide diagnostic information about the integrity of the conduction system. Sinus node dysfunction and AV conduction orders are the two major categories diagnosed and treated by invasive cardiac electrophysiology studies.[6] In sinus node dysfunction, the person has failure of sinus impulse generation or sinus impulse abnormally conducted to the atrial tissue. Invasive cardiac electrophysiology studies should be used when bradycardia cannot be clearly associated with symptoms or if clinical evidence is borderline, and in conjunction with clinical and noninvasive tests.[6] Atrioventricular conduction disorders have a clinical significance in that they block or delay conduction. Invasive cardiac-electrophysiology studies can identify the location of the site of the AV block, which is usually located within the AV node; within the His bundle (intra-Hisian); and distal to the His bundle (infra-Hisian) in the His-Purkinje system.[6] The AV conduction system can be investigated by identifying AV refractory periods; the response to medications, such as atropine or procainamide; or the response to pacing maneuvers.[6]

Electrophysiologic data is useful in predicting the risk for syncope, complete AV block, and sudden cardiac death. Electrophysiologic data is useful when symptoms are poorly correlated with bradyarrhythmias and when surface tracings cannot identify the site of the block. If patients have tachyarrhythmias or significant cardiac disease, it is important to perform ventricular stimulation with consideration of implantation of dual-chamber or biventricular ICD.[6]

CASE REPORT: BRADYARRHYTHMIAS

NC, a 59-year-of Caucasian man, presented to the emergency department with complaints of intermittent dizziness and had experienced passing out at home three times in the last month. He denied chest pain, but stated that he felt tired and noticed that performing normal activities increased his fatigue. NC's past medical history consisted of a myocardial infarction 3 years ago; a diagnosis of cardiomyopathy 1 year ago with an ejection fraction of 35%; and hypertension for 10 years. Initial assessment of vital signs revealed blood pressure at 158/92 mm Hg, pulse rate of 88 beats per minute, respiratory rate of 22 breaths per minute, temperature of 98.9°F, oxygen saturation of 98%, and cardiac monitor of sinus rhythm 84 beats per minute. Breath sounds were clear to auscultation throughout. Heart tones were audible and regular at present. There were no murmurs or gallops noted. Peripheral pulses were palpable throughout. Extremities were warm to the touch. There was no apparent distress noted. NC was admitted and transferred to the cardiovascular step down unit for further observation.

Upon admission to the cardiovascular step down unit while transferring to the bed from the stretcher, NC complained of dizziness, lightheadedness, and shortness of breath. The client was reassessed immediately with vital signs revealing blood pressure 80/40 mm Hg, pulse rate of 32 beats per minute, respiratory rate of 34 breaths per minute, temperature of 98.2°F, oxygen saturation of 86%, and cardiac monitor of sinus bradycardia with a notable 3-second pause. Rapid response was called, and NC was transferred to the cardiac intensive care unit. NC received oxygen per nasal cannula at 4 l/min, a 500 mL normal saline bolus, atropine 1mg intravenously, and a dopamine, titrate to patient's response drip at 5 mcg/kg/min. Transcutaneous pacing was started. A cardiologist referral was made. Recommendations were made for invasive cardiac electrophysiology studies to determine the feasibility of a permanent pacemaker after surface tracings could not confidently localize the site of the block.

Electrophysiologic data is helpful in diagnosis and treatment of bradyarrhythmias. The most common indications for pacemaker implantation in the United States are sinus node dysfunction followed by AV block.[7] Invasive cardiac electrophysiology studies can help predict NC's risk for syncope and sudden cardiac death. The electrophysiological studies can also identify the location of the block, response to drug therapy, response to pacing maneuvers, and validate the need for a permanent pacemaker. NC's electrophysiologic data did document the need for her to have a permanent pacemaker.

STRESS TESTING MODALITIES USING ELECTROCARDIOGRAPHY

Exercise and pharmacologic stress testing is an important electrophysiologic testing modality in the evaluation and management of patients who have known or suspected coronary heart disease and the therapeutic effects of cardiac drugs. Exercise tolerance test or stress test is noninvasive. Patients are connected to an electrocardiogram machine while exercising for 3-minute intervals. This activity puts stress on the heart and vascular system. Physical activity produces an increase in myocardial consumption, and if the supply exceeds the demand patients will experience ischemia. This electrodiagnostic test is used to document exercise-induced ischemia and identifies the risk of ischemia-induced activity.[2] If patients are unable to perform, a pharmacologic stress test may be done. Adenosine is a common drug used because it can mimic increased cardiac workload and has a short duration of action.[2] Stress testing can be performed using electrocardiography with imaging, such as with echocardiography and nuclear imaging or without imaging.[8] In nuclear imaging, patients receive an injection of a radiopharmaceutical contrast to assist in the visualization of the heart structures.[2] There are seven common types of exercise and pharmacologic stress tests that are currently in clinical use.[8] **Tables 1–7** overview these tests.[8]

CASE REPORT: EXERCISE CARDIAC STRESS TESTING

SL, a 44-year-old Caucasian man, was admitted through outpatient for an exercise cardiac stress test. He had presented 1 week ago to his primary care physician with complaints of shortness of breath, increased fatigue, chest tightness, and left-arm weakness that radiated from the shoulder area to the hand. SL's past medical history includes being overweight, a positive family history of coronary artery disease, type 2 diabetes mellitus, hypertension, cardiomyopathy, and sleep apnea.

SL's exercise cardiac stress test involved walking on the treadmill. During the exercise stress test, SL's heart rate increased to 168 beats per minute. This heart rate was maintained for 2 minutes. SL experienced slight chest discomfort, 3 out of 10, during the testing that was localized. A radiographic image of the heart was taken before and

Table 1
Treadmill exercise electrocardiography testing

Advantages	Disadvantages
Standard treadmill assessment of ischemia, functional capacity, and prognosis	Lower sensitivity
Stable results in different populations	Does not accurately localize the site or extent of myocardial ischemia

Table 2	
Exercise radionuclide myocardial perfusion imaging	
Advantages	**Disadvantages**
Accurate prognosis of extent of CAD	Cost and time commitment
Assessment of left ventricular size	Modest exposure to radiation
Assessment of myocardial viability	Artifact and quality control of trained readers

Abbreviation: CAD, coronary artery disease.

after the test was administered for comparison. When the testing was completed, the cardiologist referred the client to have a cardiac catheterization to further conclude any cardiac involvement.

A cardiac catheterization was scheduled 1week following the exercise cardiac stress test. SL was admitted through outpatient for the procedure. During the procedure, findings indicated that SL had a 90% occlusion of the right coronary artery and an 85% occlusion of the distant left circumflex artery. Angioplasty and one medicated stent to each occluded artery were performed without difficulty. SL was transferred and admitted to the cardiovascular step down unit following the procedure for overnight observation. He was discharged the following morning without notable complications.

Stress testing modalities play a diagnostic role in the treatment and management of coronary artery disease. SL's electrophysiologic testing involved exercise stress with echocardiographic images before and immediately after the peak treadmill exercise was achieved.[9] With echocardiography, cardiac function was evaluated at rest and during exercise. Risk stratification for SL and his ischemia was evaluated. Diagnostic findings provided feasibility data for referral to have a cardiac catheterization.

NERVE CONDUCTION ELECTRODIAGNOSTIC STUDIES

Nerve-conduction studies provide valuable diagnostic information to determine peripheral nervous system function, dysfunction, and disease. Electromyography (EMG or myogram) is a test that checks the health of muscles and the nerves that control the muscles. During this procedure a very thin needle electrode is inserted through the skin into the muscle. The electrode picks up this electrical activity given off by the muscles. This electrical activity is displayed on an oscilloscope.[2] After placement of the electrodes, patients are asked to contract muscles, such as their arm. The presence, size, and shape of the action potential provides information about patients' muscle ability to respond when the nerves are stimulated. There is no special preparation for a nerve conduction test. Patients are instructed to avoid using any creams or lotions on the day of the test, and that they may feel some pain and discomfort when the electrodes are inserted.[2] Patients are also instructed that the muscles may feel tender or bruised for a few days.[2]

Table 3	
Thallium versus sestamibi isotopes	
Thallium	**Sestamibi**
Detecting myocardium rest and reinjection	Superior image in obese or female patients
Assessment of pulmonary uptake	Measurement of resting left ventricular function

Table 4
Exercise radionuclide angiography

Advantages	Disadvantages
Risk stratification after myocardial infarction	Cost and limited availability
Good images with obesity and obstructive lung disease	Uses bicycle
Ejection fraction at rest and during exercise	Inaccurate with irregular heart rate Reduced specificity in females and in abnormal left ventricular function

Four primary electrophysiologic studies are used to (1) diagnose focal and generalized disorders of the peripheral nerves; (2) aid in the differentiation of primary nerve and muscle disorders; (3) classify peripheral nerve conduction abnormalities caused by axonal degeneration, demyelination, and conduction block; and (4) provide evidence-based data regarding the clinical course and efficacy of treatment.[10] A stimulating cathode (negative pole) and anode (positive pole) is placed over the nerve. Peripheral-nerve activation occurs when an electrical pulse is generated between them. Surface recording electrodes are used to record the electrical activity resulting from the nerve activation. The recording electrodes are placed over a muscle, a sensory nerve, or a cutaneous nerve distribution. Nerve-conduction studies measure three essential parameters: (1) sensory nerve action potential (SNAP) that assesses the amplitudes, areas, and configurations; (2) compound muscle action potential (CMAPs) that is generated by peripheral nerve stimulation: and (3) sensory and motor nerve conduction velocities.[8] These three measurement parameters are dependent upon the integrity of the largest myelinated fibers.

Four physiologic factors can affect nerve conduction. Nerve conduction varies in regard to specific nerves and nerve segments. For example, nerve conduction velocities are 15% to 20% faster in upper-extremity nerves than in lower-extremity nerves, and sensory conduction is 5% to 10% faster than motor conduction for each mixed nerve segment.[10] Age can affect nerve conduction because there is a negative correlation between age and evoked potential amplitude. This decline can be as much as 50% to 75% for the sensory nerve action potential, which is thought to be related to loss of nerve fibers with aging.[10] Height, weight, and gender also affect nerve conduction. There is a negative correlation between height and evoked potential amplitude especially in the lower extremity nerves. Women have faster conduction velocities than men. Body mass index affects specific nerve segments and thereby SNAP amplitudes are declined.[10]

The three main pathologic mechanisms that affect peripheral nerves are axonal degeneration, demyelination, and conduction block.[10] Nerve-conduction studies identify electropathophysiologic abnormalities that provide objective evidence of efficacy with therapy, such as when to do surgery in the carpal tunnel syndrome and

Table 5
Exercise echocardiography

Advantages	Disadvantages
Information on extent of CAD	Interpretation subjective and nonstandardized
Portable and results immediate	Poor image quality are nondiagnostic
Assesses multiple parameters	Limited number of studies

Abbreviation: CAD, coronary artery disease.

Table 6	
Pharmacologic stress testing with dipyridamole or adenosine	
Advantages	**Disadvantages**
CAD assessment without exercise	Cannot assess functional capacity
Drug side effects are rapidly reversed	ECG abnormalities less likely to occur

Abbreviation: CAD, coronary artery disease.

when to use immunosuppressive therapy in polyneuropathies.[10] The American Association of Neuromuscular and Electrodiagnostic Medicine (AANEM) recommends that nerve-conduction studies and electromyography be conducted and interpreted at the same time in the majority of test situations because the nerve conduction tests may not determine specific etiologies.[10] The AANEM published a recommended policy manual for electrodiagnostic medicine that includes a coding guide that contains ICD-9-CM codes of relevance to electrodiagnostic medicine.[11] The major complication of nerve-conduction studies is possible electrical injury from stray leakage currents. Patients in the intensive-care setting are at risk for this complication because they are attached to multiple electrical devices plugged into different power outlets. Safety procedures are necessary and the use of ground electrodes in all tests alleviate and minimize electrical leaks.[10]

ELECTRODIAGNOSTIC TESTS FOR LOW BACK PAIN

Low-back pain complaint is found in 84% of adults and is the second most common symptom complaint for physician appointments.[12] Complicated, acute low-back pain, such as nerve-impingement symptoms and fracture, requires diagnostic studies because they could have abnormal nerve function and structure. Common complaints are pain, numbness, tingling, and sensory impairment. Electrodiagnostic testing may be ordered to compliment neuroimaging. EMG is an electrodiagnostic test for evaluating and recording the activation signals of muscles. An electromyography detects the electrical potential generated by muscle cells at rest and with activity. The electromyography produces an electrograms that is read by a neurologic specialist. An electromyography can be ordered using surface electrodes or needle electrodes that are inserted through the skin into the muscle tone. Electrophysiology activity from multiple motor units is typically evaluated. A nerve-conduction test is usually done at the same time. The electromyography provides valuable diagnostic information in the diagnosis and treatment of low-back pain. For example, an EMG is sensitive in detecting disc herniations.[12] EMG is used to diagnose neuropathies and myopathies, such as peripheral neuropathy, alcoholic neuropathy, carpal tunnel syndrome, Guillain-Barré, myasthenia gravis, sciatic nerve dysfunction, and spinal stenosis.[2] Risks are minimal with

Table 7	
Dobutamine echocardiography	
Advantages	**Disadvantages**
CAD assessment without exercise	Cannot assess functional capacity
Drug side effects are rapidly reversed	ECG abnormalities less likely to occur
Detects threshold of myocardial ischemia	Labor intensive and requires experienced reader
Assessment of myocardial viability	May cause dangerous ventricular arrhythmias

Abbreviation: CAD, coronary artery disease.

an electromyography, which includes bleeding, infection at the electrode site, and trauma to the muscles that could cause false results in blood tests.[2]

CASE REPORT: NEUROPATHIES

GH, a 54-year-old man, was being evaluated by his primary care provider for a complaint of acute lower-back pain with sensory changes in bilateral lower extremities. The physical complaints included pain in the sacral area and intermittent pain and numbness experienced in the lower legs. Physical evaluation revealed that GH was moderately obese with no obvious signs of trauma or injury. Cardiac system was unremarkable and neurovascular examination was intact and with no reduction of range of motion. History included 15-year insulin-dependent diabetes mellitus that was poorly controlled. There was no history of traumatic injury to the back. X-ray reports concluded that there were no physical abnormalities on examination. Further evaluation of the lower-extremity pain indicated that there was a decrease in sensation for temperature and touch in the legs and feet bilaterally. Reflexes were unremarkable. Pulses were intact and skin color was normal. With no indication that there was a relation between GH's back pain and the lower extremities symptoms, the provider had indication to evaluate the effect that poorly controlled diabetes had on the peripheral nerves. Peripheral neuropathy affects 60% to 70% of people with insulin-dependent diabetes mellitus.[13]

A referral was made for an EMG and a nerve-conduction test. The EMG report found disc herniations and peripheral neuropathy from his complicated diabetes. GH was referred to a neurosurgeon for possible lumbar surgery and to an endocrinologist for possible insulin-pump implantation. Electrophysiological data provided valuable diagnostic data in GH's treatment.

ELECTRODIAGNOSTIC TESTING FOR SEIZURES AND EPILEPSY

Electroencephalography (EEG) is a valuable electrodiagnostic test in evaluating patients who have a possible seizure disorder. An EEG is a recording of the brain's spontaneous electrical activity over a short period of time usually 30 to 45 minutes. Electrodes are attached to the scalp with recording wires attached to a machine that records electrical impulses of brain activity. The results can be printed or displayed on a computer screen. Epileptic activity creates clear abnormalities on a standard EEG study. An example of an abnormal epileptiform activity includes interictal epileptiform discharges (IED), periodic lateralized epileptiform discharges, and generalized periodic epileptiform discharges.[13] A normal routine EEG is only 20% to 24% sensitive to IED, whereas follow-up EEG of four or more is 80% to 90% sensitive to IED.[13] The EEG duration can also affect sensitivity. An overnight EEG or mobile EEG over several days can have a higher yield of IED up to 81%.[13] Increased sensitivity also occurs when an EEG is done within 24 hours of the seizure. Specialized techniques can increase sensitivity to IED and help with classification and diagnosis of seizure or epilepsy, such as hyperventilation, photic stimulation, sleep deprivation, induced sleep, and medication withdrawal.[13] There is a wide variation in how EEGs are interpreted. A specialist is required to interpret the EEG to prevent benign patterns being misinterpreted as epileptiform.[13]

ELECTRODIAGNOSTIC STUDY FOR OBSTRUCTIVE SLEEP APNEA IN ADULTS

Laboratory hallmarks of obstructive sleep apnea in adults are periodic apneas and hypopneas during sleep, episodic flow-limited breaths, and multiple arousals during sleep.[14] Daytime somnolence is a common feature. Obstructive sleep apnea is usually suspected when patients have excessive daytime sleepiness with witnessed apneas and snoring.[15] A polysomnography is the gold standard diagnostic test for obstructive sleep apnea.[15] Patients sleep while connected to numerous monitoring devices and a technologist records physiologic variables. The following list overviews the physiologic variables[15]:

- Sleep stages (Electroencephalographic activity [EEG], eye movements [electro-oculograms], and electromyographic activity [EMG] are recorded to identify the stages of sleep.)[15]
- Respiratory sleep (Indices are derived from polysomnograhic data that includes apnea index, apnea-hypopnea index, respiratory index, and snoring.)[15]
- Oxygen saturation (Pulse oximetry is used to monitor arterial oxyhemoglobin saturation.)[15]
- Electrocardiogram (Detection of arrhythmias during sleep.)[15]
- Body position (Position sensor is used to document patients' position and changes in position.)[15]
- Limb movements (An EMG of the anterior tibialis of both legs is monitored to identify limb movements during sleep.)[15]

Complications of a polysomnography are rare. The most common complication is skin irritation caused by adhesive used to attach electrodes to patients. Inconveniences are reported, such as difficulty sleeping in the laboratory setting, strange surroundings, discomfort related to the monitoring equipment, and time needed to spend the night at the sleep clinic.[15] Education of patients before a polysomnography include advisement not to consume alcohol or caffeine and to continue their usual medications on the night of the PSG, including sleep aids.[15]

SUMMARY

This article overviews electrodiagnostic tests that provide evidence-based data in the treatment and management of abnormalities in nerves and muscles. There is a focused review on cardiac tests, nerve-conduction tests, low-back pain tests, seizure and epilepsy tests, and obstructive sleep apnea electrodiagnostic tests. Case reports demonstrate how these electrophysiologic tests can provide specific data about the location and underlying causative factors of abnormalities in the nerves and muscles that routine diagnostic tests cannot differentiate.

REFERENCES

1. Sole ML, Klein D, Moseley M. Cardiovascular alterations. In: Iannuzzi M, Hlersi J, editors. Introduction to critical care nursing. 5th edition. St Louis (MO): Saunders Elsevier; 2009. p. 317–69.
2. Hoch DB. Medline plus. Medical encyclopedia: electromyography. Available at: http://www.nlm.nih.gov/medlineplus.print/ency/article/003929.htm. Accessed May 2, 2009.
3. Podrid PJ, Ganz L, Knight BP, et al, editors. Overview of invasive cardiac electrophysiology studies. UpToDate. Available at: http://www.update.com/home/index.html. Accessed April 4, 2009.
4. Knight BP, Olshanky B, Blaustein RD, editors. Electrophysiologic cardiac mapping: use in specific arrhythmias. UpToDate. Available at: http://www.update.com/home/index.html. Accessed April 4, 2009.

5. Porid PJ, Zimetbaum PJ, Blaustein RO. Invasive cardiac electrophysiology studies: tachyarrhythmias. UpToDate. Available at: http://www.update.com./home/index.html. Accessed April 4, 2009.

6. Germano JJ, Zimetbaum PJ, Blaustein RO, editors. Invasive cardiac electrophysiology studies: bradyarrhythmias. UpToDate. Available at: http://www.update.com./home/index.html. Accessed April 4, 2009.

7. Hayes DL, Gantz LI, Blaustein RD, editors. Indications for permanent cardiac pacing. UpToDate. Available at: http://www.uptodate.com.home/index.html. Accessed March 14, 2009.

8. Weiner DA, Manning WJ, Iskandrian AE, et al, editors. Advantages and limitations of different stress testing. UpToDate. Available at: http://www.uptodate.com.home/index.html. Accessed March 14, 2007.

9. Schiller NB, Ren X, Ristow B, et al, editors. Protocols for stress echocardiography. UpToDate. Available at: http://www.uptodate.com.home/index.html. Accessed March 14, 2009.

10. Horowitz SH, Shefner JM, Dashe JH, editors. Nerve conduction studies: basic principles. UpToDate. Available at: http://www.uptodate.com.home/index.html. Accessed April 4, 2009.

11. American Association of Neuromuscular & Electrodiagnostic Medicine. Recommended policy for electrodiagnostic medicine. Available at: http://uptodate.com.home/index/html. Accessed April 4, 2009.

12. Staiger TO, Gatewood M, Wipf JE, et al, editors. Diagnostic testing for low back pain. UpToDate. Available at: http://www.uptodate.com/home/index.html. Accessed April 4, 2009.

13. Hirsh LJ, Hiba A, Pedley TA, et al, editors. Electroencephalography (EEG) in the diagnosis of seizures and epilepsy. UpToDate. Available at: http://www.uptodate.com/home/index.html. Accessed April 4, 2009.

14. Hirsch LJ, Anif H, Pealey TA, et al, editors. Clinical presentation and diagnosis of obstructive sleep apnea in adults. UpToDate. Available at: http://www.uptodate.com/home/index.html. Accessed April 4, 2009.

15. Millgan RP, Kramer NR. Polysomnography in obstructive sleep apnea in adults. UpToDate. Available at: http://www.uptodate.com/home/index.html. Accessed April 4, 2009.

Endoscopy: A Guide for the Registered Nurse

Sandra R. Scholten, MSN, FNP-BC

KEYWORDS

- Endoscopy • Gastrointestinal procedures
- Nursing implications • Patient education
- Complications

As an invasive procedure, endoscopic studies require patient care and considerations that are very similar to minor surgical procedures. There are some general guidelines that are applicable to all endoscopic procedures, and there are special considerations that are dictated by the specific endoscopic procedure. It is important for the critical care nurse to understand the procedures because the differences and similarities of each procedure guide nursing actions to affect the best patient outcomes.

ENDOSCOPY: WHAT IS IT?

To enhance the critical care nurse's perspective of the impact of the test on the patient, there is foundational knowledge about endoscopy that must be considered. Endoscopy is a procedure designed to view the interior body with use of a flexible optical tube called an "endoscope."[1] The type of procedure is generally named for the area of the body that needs to be examined.[2] With the aid of endoscopy providers are able to view several different regions of the body including the upper and lower gastrointestinal (GI) tract, pancreas and bile ducts, joints, and lungs, and evaluate blood flow with the addition of ultrasound. Endoscopy can be used for early detection, management, and treatment of diseases. During the procedure it is possible to collect tissue needed for biopsies, remove potential precancerous lesions, stop bleeding, reduce the size of tumors, place stents, reverse a volvulus, and remove foreign bodies. Endoscopy procedures are generally safe and have a complication rate of only 0.1% to 0.2% and an even lower mortality rate of 0.03%. Significant complications related to the procedure and those that are caused by the anesthesia during endoscopy include respiratory depression, aspiration, perforation, and bleeding.[1]

This article includes a summary of the common endoscopic procedures and provides information about possible postprocedure complications. An in-depth look

Vanderbilt School of Nursing, 345 Frist Hall, 461 21st Avenue South, Nashville, TN 37240, USA
E-mail address: Sandra.r.scholten@vanderbilt.edu

Crit Care Nurs Clin N Am 22 (2010) 19–32
doi:10.1016/j.ccell.2009.10.002
0899-5885/10/$ – see front matter © 2010 Elsevier Inc. All rights reserved.
ccnursing.theclinics.com

at GI endoscopy studies is included along with nursing considerations. After reading this article the registered nurse should be able to describe various endoscopic procedures, common complications, nursing interventions, and patient education important to each study.

UPPER GI STUDIES
Endoscopic Retrograde Cholangiopancreatography

Endoscopic retrograde cholangiopancreatography (ERCP) is a procedure designed to evaluate problems associated with the liver, gallbladder, bile ducts, and pancreatic ducts.[3] The endoscope is moved though the esophagus and stomach until it reaches the duodenum. Once the endoscope is in place, evaluation of the common bile duct, the hepatic bile ducts, and the pancreatic ducts is possible. During the procedure contrast dye is inserted in the ducts and radiographs are taken to evaluate the organs and to detect any abnormalities, such as stones, tumors, strictures, or injury.[4]

Before the procedure the patient is kept "nothing by mouth" (NPO) for 6 hours.[5] Consent for the procedure should be obtained because it is an invasive procedure requiring sedation. Nurses should also remember to ask the patient about allergies specifically to iodine, shellfish, and contrast media before the procedure because of risk of anaphylactic reactions to contrast dye.[6]

Complications of ERCP include pancreatitis, bleeding, perforation, cholangitis, cholecystitis, and cardiopulmonary events. ERCP-induced pancreatitis is defined as "new or worsened abdominal pain and a serum amylase that is 3 or more times the upper limits of normal 24 hours after the procedure that requires at least 2 days of hospitalization."[7] Reportedly, studies have found that pancreatitis was the most commonly reported complication with an occurrence rate of 1% to 7%.[7] Other researchers have studied post-ERCP complications and found similar results. Pancreatitis was the most commonly reported complication. Most cases were treatable; however, some did result in death.[8] More recently, studies have been done to determine to what extent nafamostat mesylate, a synthetic serine protease inhibitor, prevents ERCP-related pancreatitis. Results are promising but more research using this substance must be completed before it is recommended as a standard of care.[9]

Bleeding may occur, especially if a sphincterotomy is performed during the ERCP. The risk of bleeding is low (0.76%–2%) with severe bleeding requiring blood transfusion even lower (0.1%–0.5%).[7] Some studies report bleeding rates to be 2 in 39 patients.[8] Signs of bleeding may include melena, hematochezia, or hematemesis.[7]

Another rare but serious complication is perforation. Perforation occurs in 0.3% to 0.6% of ERCP cases.[6] These perforations can be fatal.[7] If a perforation is recognized and treated quickly patients recover without surgical intervention. Billroth II partial gastrectomy, the performance of a sphincterotomy, the intramural injection of contrast, duration of procedure, biliary stricture dilation, and sphincter of Oddi dysfunction impose risks for perforation. Signs of perforation may include pain, fever, leukocytosis, pneumomediastinum and subcutaneous emphysema, and pneumothorax.[6]

Cholangitis, an infection of biliary tract, and cholecystitis, inflammation of the gallbladder, are two possible postprocedure complications occurring in 1% or less and 0.2% to 0.5%, respectively. Signs of cholangitis include fever, abdominal pain, and yellowing of the skin and sclera.[10] Signs of cholecystitis include epigastic pain, upper abdominal pain radiating to the right scapula, nausea, vomiting, and fever.[11]

Cardiopulmonary complications (arrhythmias, aspiration, hypoventilation caused by medications) although rare, occurring less than 1%, can be fatal.[7] This type of complication is rare and is probably caused by sedation, longer procedure times, prone positioning, advanced age, and comorbid diseases.[6] Although advanced age is usually included as a risk factor for complication of procedures, there is some indication that ERCP in patients over 90 years of age is safe. In the elderly, the major risks for this procedure are associated with the sedation required.[12]

Other complications of ERCP include ileus; antibiotic-related diarrhea; hepatic abscess formation; pneumothorax; pneumomediastinum; perforation of colonic diverticular; duodenal hematoma; portal venous air; and impaction of therapeutic devices, such as stone retrieval baskets.[7] Although there are a variety of possible complications after ERCP, the rates are relatively low. It is important for the critical care nurse to monitor vital signs, perform frequent head to toe assessments, and report changes that may indicate a complication. Through continuous observation and prompt intervention negative patient outcomes can be minimized.

Esophagogastroduodenoscopy

Esophagogastroduodenoscopy (EGD) is an invasive upper GI endoscopic procedure. During this procedure an endoscope is inserted into the mouth and passed through the esophagus and stomach until the duodenum is reached. EGD allows the provider to visualize, photograph, biopsy, cauterize, or inject any abnormalities between the mouth and duodenum. Unlike ERCP, contrast dye is not used during this procedure.

EGD can aid in the diagnosis of several disorders including bleeding, esophageal and gastric varices, polyps, tumors, ulcers, esophagitis, gastritis, esophageal stenosis, and gastroesophageal reflux.[4] This procedure may be performed to evaluate complaints of abdominal pain, nausea, vomiting, and painful swallowing. EGD has even been useful in diagnosing Crohn's disease.[3]

Complications of EGD are minimal but those that occur are most typically infection, bleeding, perforation, and cardiopulmonary events. In most cases, medications do not need to be discontinued before the procedure unless tissue removal is anticipated.[13]

In preparation for the procedure the patient should be NPO for about 6 hours. Patients should be informed that they will remain NPO until their gag reflex returns after the procedure. Informed consent should be obtained. Explain to the patient that an intravenous catheter is placed to give sedation during the procedure. Topical anesthetic is sprayed in the back of the patient's throat to numb the area where the tube is inserted. A bite block is used to prevent damage to the endoscope and make it easier for the tube to pass through the mouth. The procedure lasts approximately 5 to 30 minutes (longer if any interventions need to be performed) and it usually takes about 1 hour for recovery. After the patient has recovered (alert, oriented, and ambulatory) from the sedation he or she is allowed to leave with an escort to drive them home. Instructions regarding diet, activity, and monitoring for complications should be given to the patient. A follow-up appointment should be made and given to the patient before departure.[13]

Capsule Endoscopy

With this technology, the small intestine can be visualized in a minimally invasive way. The patient is instructed to swallow a capsule (11 × 30 mm) sized camera.[14] The capsule not only contains the camera but also a light bulb, battery, and radio transmitter. As it travels through the GI system, thousands of images are captured and transmitted to a device that the patient wears on his or her belt. The images are later downloaded to a computer for review. The capsule should pass through the GI tract with feces.[3,15]

Capsule endoscopy is not an option for patients who have strictures, known bowel obstruction,[3] tumors,[15] and fistulas because of the risk of bowel obstruction.[14] Other problems that may be encountered with this method of endoscopy are issues relating to transit. If the capsule is moving to quickly through the intestines, the images may be blurry or hard to decipher. If the camera is moving too slowly, several pictures of the same area are taken and the battery life (about 6 hours) is depleted before reaching the end of the small intestine.[14] Even if clear pictures are obtained, it can also be difficult to pinpoint the exact location a problem. Sifting through several thousand photos can be very time consuming and tedious for providers.

There are several aspects of patient preparation that help to ensure effective results. The bowel must be cleared so images of the intestine are not obstructed. The patient should not eat or drink anything for up to 12 hours before swallowing the camera.[16] For specifics on bowel preparation and dosing schedules see **Table 1**. Two hours after swallowing the camera, the patient is allowed to drink clear liquids. Four hours after ingestion of the camera the patient can eat a light meal. Although it is acceptable for the patient to return to normal activities and work after swallowing the camera,[14] patients should be told not to participate in vigorous activities, such as running and jumping. The nurse should also remember to ask the patient about all medications he or she is taking including over-the-counter medications, iron, and aspirin.[16] If the patient has taken medications that may increase the risk of bleeding or obstruct the view of the intestinal walls, notify the provider ordering the test.

Capsule endoscopy is helpful in diagnosing angiodysplasias, small intestinal tumors, Crohn disease,[15] and celiac disease.[14] It can be used to evaluate abdominal pain, anemia, indigestion,[15] and erosions.[14]

Although rare, the most common complication of capsule endoscopy is obstruction. The patient presents with complaints of bloating, abdominal pain, and vomiting after the procedure. Educate the patient to report signs of obstruction along with fever, trouble swallowing, and chest pain.[16]

Endoscopic Ultrasound

Endoscopic ultrasound (EUS) is a minimally invasive procedure that allows visualization of the intestinal walls with great detail by combining endoscopy and ultrasound.[17] An ultrasound probe is placed on the endoscope and provides valuable information about tissues that lay deep within the intestines. This procedure is useful in evaluating fistulas of the rectum and for obtaining biopsies.[3] Through this procedure, diagnosticians are able to stage cancers (lung, esophageal, gastric, rectal, and pancreatic) and examine the surrounding tissues and lymph nodes for metastasis; find stones in the common bile duct; evaluate masses and enlarged stomach folds; diagnose disease of the pancreas; and collect fluid and tissue samples. EUS has been instrumental in the diagnosis of several conditions including Barrett esophagus, neuroendocrine tumors, common bile duct stones, gastric cancer, esophageal cancer, lung cancer, pancreatic cancer, pancreatitis, cystic neoplasms of the pancreas, rectal cancer, rectal fistulas, smooth muscle tumors, and enlarged lymph nodes.[17]

EUS can be an upper or lower GI tract procedure. For upper GI tests the patient needs to be NPO for at least 6 hours before the test. For a lower GI tract examination the patient needs to be on a clear liquid diet and take one of the bowel preparations indicated in **Table 1**.[15]

For the upper EUS, the patient's throat is sprayed with numbing medications and sedation is required. When performing lower EUS sedation may or may not be used. The tube is moved through the digestive tract with the patient lying on his or

Table 1
Dosing schedule for lower endoscopy bowel preparation

| Type | Day Before Procedure | | Day of Procedure | | How Long | Special Consideration |
	Amount	Frequency	Amount	Frequency		
PEG-ELS	240 mL	q 10 min			Feces are clear or entire volume consumed	No solid food for 2 h before beginning preparation; only clear liquids day of procedure
2-L PEG-ELS + bisacodyl	240 mL	q 10 min			Total volume consumed	Take 6 bisacodyl before beginning preparation; only clear liquids the day of procedure
2-L PEG-ELS + ascorbic acid	240 mL	q 15 min	240 mL	q 15 min	Total volume consumed	Start 1 h before light supper on the day before procedure and follow with 480 mL of clear liquid; the remaining solution should be drank either 1.5 h after the first half or on the morning of the procedure
Sodium phosphate 90 mL	45 mL	x1	45 mL	x1	Total volume consumed	Dilute each glass with 240 mL of water and follow with 480 mL of clear liquids; take each dose 10 to 12 h apart
Sodium phosphate tablets	4 tablets	q 15 min	4 tablets	q 15 min	20 tablets night before procedure; take remaining pills on day of procedure	Followed by 240 mL of water; on day of procedure start taking pills 3–5 h before procedure

Data from A-Rahim YI, Falchuk M. Bowel preparation for colonoscopy. UpToDate 2009. Available at: http://www.uptodate.com/online/content/topic.do?topic Key=gi_endos/6324&view=print. Accessed April 23, 2009.

her left side. Depending on the extent of tissue needing to be examined the procedure lasts 10 to 45 minutes.[16]

Complications of upper EUS include bleeding, adverse affects caused by anesthetics, aspiration, infection, and perforation. Common complaints after the procedure are a sore throat and bloating. Patients should be told to alert the critical care nurse if they feel sore throat and bloating so that measures can be taken to alleviate symptoms.[16]

Double Balloon Endoscopy

The double balloon endoscopy is a relatively new procedure used to visualize the small intestine. The endoscope can be inserted either orally or rectally. It can be used to remove video capsules that have not passed through the GI tract successfully or to diagnose Meckel diverticulum. This procedure can be used to detect injuries to the small intestinal wall and diaphragm, ulceration associated with Crohn disease, polyps that have caused intussusception, hematomas related to anticoagulant therapy, lymphoma, tumors, Gorham disease, diverticulosis, eosinophilic jejunitis, and familial adenomatous polyposis. The test is usually performed after failed attempts at colonoscopy. It has also been able to detect tumors that might not have been identified through the use of wireless capsule endoscopy.[18]

During the procedure the endoscope is advanced with the use of two balloons that allow the tube to advance through the small intestine, much like a worm. This technique allows the provider to harvest tissue samples, perform hemostasis, perform balloon dilatation, place a stent, remove polyps, or remove mucosa.[18]

Complications after the procedure are similar to complications associated with a colonoscopy or sigmoidoscopy. Serious complications include pancreatitis, bleeding, and perforation. Bleeding has been associated with one reported death after this procedure. Hyperamylasemia has also been reported without other signs of pancreatitis.[18]

LOWER GI STUDIES
Bowel Preparation for Lower GI Endoscopic Procedures

To prepare the bowel for a lower GI endoscopic procedure the gut has to be cleared of all fecal matter. This enables the endoscopist to clearly visualize the intestinal wall for lesions, polyps, source of bleeding, and tumors. There are several types of bowel preparation that can be divided into two distinct categories: high volume or low volume. The high-volume preparations include polyethylene glycol–electrolyte lavage (PEG-ELS) solutions. The lower-volume preparations include sodium phosphate, magnesium citrate, and saline laxatives. All bowel preparations have similar efficacy; however, some are tolerated better than others. The ordering provider and nurse administering the medications, however, also have to be aware of special considerations with each type of preparation and patient population.[19]

The PEG-ELS solutions come in a 2- or 4-L concentration. This type of solution is osmotically balanced,[19] meaning there is no need for passage of liquid into or out of the gut to aid with expulsion of contents.[20] These solutions are able to clear the GI tract because the solution cannot be absorbed by the patient's body.

Originally, PEG-ELS solutions were only made in a 4-L solution and they were unpalatable because of the salty taste. Manufacturers reformulated the preparation as a sulfate free to reduce the saltiness and provided flavoring, which was more accepted by patients. They have also developed a 2-L preparation that incorporated either bisacodyl or ascorbic acid. The lower volume was also appreciated by patients. All of the aforementioned preparations have comparable results regarding bowel evacuation but patients prefer the smaller volume and sulfate free solutions.[19]

There are similar side effects of all bowel preparations but the PEG-ELS solutions have been linked to less fluid and electrolyte shifts than the low-volume solutions. Side effects for the high-volume preparations include dehydration and resulting orthostatic hypotension, nausea, and vomiting. Despite the relative safety of this preparation type there are reasons that the high-volume solution should not be given to certain patients. It should not be given to anyone with a diagnosis of ileus, gastric retention, bowel perforation, GI obstruction, or severe colitis.[19,21] Additionally, patients with impaired swallowing should not be given this preparation orally, but should receive it by nasogastric tube.[21]

There are several aspects of patient education that the nurse should consider when teaching patients about this type of bowel preparation. Emphasize the importance of drinking all of the solution to ensure that adequate bowel clearing is achieved. Some providers may recommend continuing ingestion of the solution only until feces become watery and clear.[21] If this is the case, be sure to tell the patient how to evaluate for this change. Patients are who are well informed are more motivated to take part in their care.

High-volume preparations may be chosen for patients at risk for fluid and electrolyte imbalance. These patients have diagnoses including renal disease, congestive heart failure, liver disease, or any type of preprocedure electrolyte imbalance.[21] Providing information about common side effects is essential and helps alleviate patient anxiety when side effects occur.

In cases of nausea, the patient should try drinking the solution slower or take antinausea medications (compazine or metoclopramide). To mask the unpleasant taste patients can refrigerate the solution; suck on lemon wedges between sips; or add sugar-free powdered flavor enhancers, such as Crystal Light (a flavor that does not add red dye to the preparation), or lemon juice.[21]

The small-volume solutions used for bowel preparation are hyperosmotic and draw fluid into the intestinal tract. These solutions have been found to be well tolerated by patients and have similar efficacy regarding bowel cleaning but have the potential to cause serious electrolyte imbalance and intravascular volume depletion.[19]

Saline laxatives are a type of small-volume bowel preparation. The mechanism of action of saline laxatives occurs when magnesium or phosphate ions cause the retention of water in the small intestine, which in turn stimulates stretch receptors and increases peristalsis. Types of saline laxatives include sodium picosulfate and magnesium citrate, which is used in the United Kingdom[19]; sodium phosphate solution, which is currently banned by the Food and Drug Administration in the United States; and sodium phosphate tablets, which carry a black box warning from the Food and Drug Administration for renal toxicity and renal failure.[21]

Sodium phosphate formulations are saline laxatives and are available as a 90-mL solution, 80-mL solution, 40 tablets, or 32 tablets. The tablet formulations were introduced more recently. The first tablet form of sodium phosphate (40 tablets) contained a substance called "microcrystalline cellulose." Although this formulation is tolerable it has been found to limit the endoscopist's view of the colon. A newer tablet form (32 tablets) does not include the microcrystalline cellulose ingredient. These newer choices have been tolerated and efficacious. They have comparable side effects as the PEG-ELS including abdominal distention, nausea, vomiting, headache, anal discomfort, and pain.[19]

Patients with renal disease, liver disease, and chronic heart failure should not take sodium phosphate solutions or tablets because of the high potential of electrolyte imbalance.[19] Other contraindications are a glomerular filtration rate less than 50 and preprocedure electrolyte imbalance. Patients taking diuretics, angiotensin-converting enzyme inhibitors, angiotensin-receptor blockers, or nonsteroidal anti-inflammatory drugs should be monitored closely because of the risk for electrolyte imbalances. The critical care nurse should be vigilant to potential tonic-clonic seizures, and the development of inflammatory bowel diseases when the patient is given these preparations. These preparations should be given very cautiously to the elderly because age-related changes to kidney function predispose this population to electrolyte imbalance. Because lesions may be caused from sodium phosphate it is advised for use if the patient has confirmed or suspected inflammatory bowel disease or diarrhea of unknown origin.[21]

Magnesium citrate is a hyperosmotic solution and works like sodium phosphate by drawing fluid into the intestines. It can be used in conjunction to PEG-ELS solutions to improve bowel clearing.[19] Because it is a hyperosmotic solution it can be expected to have the same electrolyte disturbance potential, contraindications, and side effects as other small-volume preparations. Despite its limitations in certain patient populations excellent results have been reported.[21]

Regardless of the type of preparation used instructions regarding diet, medications, and adequate patient hydration should always be given. Patients must have a clear understanding of the dietary modifications required for testing. Tests are most effective when the patient is involved and understands expectations. The patient is often on a clear liquid diet (water, clear broth, coffee, tea, ice, gelatin, and fruit juice) the day before the procedure; however, they should be told to avoid red liquids because they mimic areas of bleeding.[21] Patients can typically consume the clear liquid diet up to 2 to 5 hours before the procedure.[19,21]

Most medications are safe for the patient to take before the procedure. Some should be stopped up to 7 days before the procedure (aspirin, nonsteroidal anti-inflammatory drugs, anticoagulants, and iron). Nurses should remember to ask patients if they have taken any of these types of medication during the week before the procedure and if so, notify the physician performing the procedure.[19]

The potential for dehydration is present with all forms of bowel preparation, but can be minimized by drinking fluids often while taking the bowel preparation. The patient should be encouraged to drink carbohydrate-electrolyte rehydration solution. If the patient does not make a conscious effort to drink large amounts of fluids he or she is at risk for orthostatic hypotension and consequences of dehydration.[19] **Table 1** summarizes the dosing schedule for lower GI bowel preparations and **Table 2** lists the types of bowel preparations and associated brand or generic names.

Colonoscopy

A colonoscopy is performed to examine the entire length of the colon and at times, the end of the ileum.[2,3] The endoscope is introduced through the anus and passed through the intestines. Many people are familiar with colonoscopies because they are used to screen for colon cancer for those over 50, or earlier if there is a family history of cancer. This test can also be used to evaluate complaints of bleeding, diarrhea, iron deficiency anemia, weight loss, and abdominal pain. The procedure might be used in cases of abnormal barium enema results or if the patient has a history of colon polyps or ulcerative colitis. It can also be used for management of Crohn disease and ulcerative colitis.[4,22] The procedure usually takes 20 to 60 minutes.[22]

Bowel preparation is typically the most cumbersome part of the colonoscopy. Patients have dietary restrictions and are given a strict regimen to follow to provide adequate bowel cleansing. An assessment of the patient's medication regimen should

Table 2
Names of bowel preparations

Type	Name	Specifications
PEG-ELS	Golytely	
	Nulytely	Sodium sulfate free version of Golytely
	Colyte	
	Colyte-Flavored	Flavored version of Colyte
2-L PEG-ELS + bisacodyl	HalfLytely	Nulytely + bisacodyl
2-L PEG-ELS + ascorbic acid	MoviPrep	
Sodium phosphate	Fleet Phospho-Soda	Comes in ginger-lemon flavor or unflavored. Banned by Food and Drug Administration
Sodium phosphate tablets	Visicol	
	OsmoPrep TM	Microcrystalline cellulose -free formulation. Black box warning for renal toxicity
Combination	Fleet prep kit	Includes sodium phosphate, flavored castor oil, and bisacodyl Comes in a suppository or enema form
Sodium picosulfate	Picoprep-3	

Data from A-Rahim YI, Falchuk M. Bowel preparation for colonoscopy. UpToDate 2009. Available at: http://www.uptodate.com/online/content/topic.do?topicKey=gi_endos/6324&view=print. Accessed April 23, 2009.

be done before the procedure. In general, it is advised that patients stop taking medications with anticoagulant properties (aspirin, Coumadin, nonsteroidal anti-inflammatory drugs) and iron for 1 to 2 weeks before the procedure.[22]

Complications of colonoscopies included peritonitis, perforation, septicemia, diaphragmatic hernias, adverse effects from sedation, bleeding, and phlebitis. Peritonitis is a particular risk for patients with ascites. For the patient with ascites, antibiotics are recommended for prophylaxis.[23] Although rare, perforations that occur during this procedure are particularly serious.[24] Some reports indicate colonoscopic retroflexion can result in rectal perforation. Although most patients recover without further invasive intervention, some may require surgical intervention. Septicemia can occur after colonoscopy but may be attributed to other causes rather than to the procedure itself.[25] Diaphragmatic hernias before 1999[26] were not known to be complications of colonoscopies. Bleeding is a possibility after tissue removal. Any patient requiring intravenous fluids and medication could suffer from phlebitis, which occurs because of inflammation to the vein.[22]

Like the other lower GI procedures, the patient lays on his or her left side during the procedure. The patient receives relaxing and pain medications before the procedure, and is assessed throughout the procedure for pain and anxiety. Once inserted, the scope is advanced through the rectum and images of the colon are shown on a monitor for the provider to view. Should a polyp be encountered, it can be removed during the procedure. Air and fluid can also be sprayed into the gut and withdrawn. The patient may a feel temporary bloating, cramping, or abdominal discomfort because of the air or fluid. It is important to tell the patient to expel gas when needed during the procedure and not to be embarrassed.[22]

When patients receive preprocedure information they are less anxious and have a higher threshold for pain. Nursing interventions that may help patients experience less pain and anxiety include calm talk, explaining reasons for pain, and the cause of symptoms. Tell the patient when to expect pain during the procedure. Keeping patients in a warm, dry, and relaxed pose may also be helpful. In some cases, the patient may hyperventilate. In these cases, assist and instruct the patient to breath into a paper bag. Reducing environmental stimuli by darkening and calming the room, using humor, assisting in position changes, massaging or touching the patient, and using breathing techniques might help reduce pain and anxiety.[27]

After the procedure the patient should be monitored until the anesthetics have been metabolized and the patient is alert and ambulatory. The patient will be drowsy and will need an escort home. Although the patient is encouraged not to go to work after the procedure, once home he or she can resume a regular diet. The patient should be instructed to notify a health care provider if severe abdominal pain is encountered; the patient's abdomen becomes distended; or if vomiting, fever, or rectal bleeding develops.[22]

Nursing activities relating to colonoscopies include ensuring that the provider performing the scope has explained the procedure, risks, and benefits, and then obtaining a signed consent. The nurse also starts an intravenous catheter; gives medications; monitors for changes in vital signs (before, during, and after the procedure); administers oxygen if needed; and educates the patient about follow-up activity and symptoms that should be reported. It is important for the nurse to recognize signs of complications and promptly intervene. For example, a change in blood pressure and heart rate may indicate bleeding, complaints of abdominal pain could indicate a perforation, and fever and chills may be present if perforation has occurred.[22]

Flexible Sigmoidoscopy

Flexible sigmoidoscopy is a procedure that allows for the visualization of the rectum, sigmoid colon, and proximal colon.[4] This procedure is performed to evaluate symptoms of bright red rectal bleeding, discharge, protrusions, pain,[4] and diarrhea.[28] It can be used to screen for colon cancer, evaluate the bowel after pelvic radiation, and to manage colitis. Flexible sigmoidoscopy has also proved helpful when used in conjunction with barium enemas.[28] The procedure can be used to diagnose tumors, polyps, and diverticular disease. Biopsies can be taken during the procedure if needed.[4]

Bowel preparation is necessary (see **Table 1**). Medications that should be discontinued before the procedure include medications with anticoagulant properties and iron. Iron has a propensity to adhere to the wall of the colon.[21] Because most endoscopy studies are considered invasive, an informed consent is warranted.

During the procedure the patient is positioned on his or her left side. Intravenous sedation is usually not required.[28] The endoscope is lubricated and then advanced through the rectum and anal sphincter.[1] The duration of a flexible sigmoidoscopy is about 5 to 15 minutes. Patients should be instructed that while air is injected and the scope is advanced they may feel some abdominal cramping. The patient does not feel pain if a biopsy is taken because the colon lining is not able to sense pain.[28]

The most common complications after a flexible sigmoidoscopy are bleeding from biopsy or polyp removal, perforation, and peritonitis. Patients should be instructed to notify the nurse or health care provider if they develop signs of a complication (abdominal pain, distended abdomen, vomiting, fever, and bleeding). Typically, the procedure is tolerated without major complications and the patient is able to resume activities of daily living and a regular diet once returning home.[22]

Table 3
Nursing consideration for gastrointestinal endoscopy

Test	Upper/Lower GI	Nursing Consideration Before Procedure	Nursing Consideration After Procedure
Endoscopic retrograde cholangiopancreatography	Upper GI	Keep patient NPO Allergy to contrast dye Consent needed Inquire about medications	Monitor vital signs Perform frequent physical assessments Report changes to doctor
Esophagogastroduodenoscopy	Upper GI	Keep patient NPO Allergy to contrast Start IV Inquire about medications	Keep NPO until gag reflex returns Follow-up instructions and appointment
Capsule endoscopy	Upper GI	Keep pt NPO Inquire about medications Obtain informed consent	Clear liquids 2 h after swallowing Light meal 4 h after swallowing Watch for bloating, abdominal pain, vomiting, fever, trouble swallowing, and chest pain
Endoscopic ultrasound	Upper GI or lower GI	Keep patient NPO if upper Clear liquid diet if lower Start IV Obtain informed consent Inquire about medications	Keep NPO until gag reflex returns Watch for bleeding, adverse affects caused by anesthetics, aspiration, infection, and perforation
Double balloon endoscopy	Upper GI or lower GI		
Colonoscopy	Lower GI	Inquire about medications Ask if patient completed preparation Start IV Tell patient to expel gas as needed Obtain signed consent form	Monitor vital signs Perform frequent physical assessments Report changes to doctor Administer oxygen prn
Flexible sigmoidoscopy	Lower GI	Inquire about medications Ask if patient completed preparation Start IV Tell patient to expel gas as needed Obtain signed consent form	Monitor vital signs Perform frequent physical assessments Report changes to doctor Administer oxygen prn

Box 1
Websites for information about endoscopic examinations

- American Society of Gastrointestinal Endoscopy Web site (http://www.asge.org/PatientInfo Index.aspx?id=1022).
- National Institute of Health (http://www.nih.gov/)
- National Library of Medicine (http://www.nlm.nih.gov/)
- American Society of Gastrointestinal Endoscopy (http://www.asge.org/)
- The National Digestive Disease Information Clearinghouse (http://digestive.niddk.nih.gov/)

Anoscopy

Anoscopy is an endoscopic procedure very similar to sigmoidoscopy. It can be used to find polyps, inflammation, diverticular disease, bleeding, and hemorrhoids. The difference between the procedures is that the endoscope is inserted a much shorter distance (2 in) and a digital rectal examination is performed before insertion of the endoscope. Because of the short distance into the lower GI tract there is no bowel preparation needed.[29]

Proctoscopy

A proctoscopy is also use to evaluate similar lower GI complaints. The patient should complete a bowel preparation and only consume clear liquids before the procedure. Immediately before insertion of the endoscope a digital rectal examination is performed. A proctoscope is then inserted into the rectum to assess the lining and identify abnormalities. Biopsies can be taken during the procedure. Positioning and complications of other lower GI scopes are the same as with proctoscopy.[29]

SEDATION RELATED TO ENDOSCOPIES

There are several options with regard to sedation during endoscopic procedures. As with any medication the patient is taking, it is the nurse's responsibility to know common side effects and be able to carefully monitor for those side effects. Important aspects that warrant monitoring while a patient is recovering from sedation include respiratory rate and pattern, oxygen saturation, level of consciousness, blood pressure, and heart rate. Each sedative used for procedural sedation has its own advantages and disadvantages for use. There are also patient risk factors, such as age, obesity, comorbities, and sleep apnea, which impact the potential adverse effects of sedation during these procedures.[30]

SUMMARY

When caring for a patient undergoing an endoscopy, the nurse should remember to obtain information regarding allergies and past medical history before the procedure. A signed consent must be completed and education regarding the specific procedure should be explained to the patient before the procedure begins. During the procedure the nurse is responsible for administering medications, monitoring vital signs, and reporting significant changes. During the recovery period it is crucial that frequent assessments are performed with particular attention to the abdominal region. Other parameters that must be monitored include temperature, vital signs, and indications of bleeding. Changes in patient status and patient complaints may be indicative of a complication and should be reported promptly. Nurses are also instrumental in providing instructions including activity, diet, and follow-up appointments to the patient before discharge. For a summary of nursing considerations see **Table 3**. **Box 1** provides some current Web sites to find additional information about endoscopic testing.

REFERENCES

1. Diagnostic and therapeutic GI procedures. In: Beers MH, Porter RS, Jones TV, et al, editors. Merck manual. 18th edition. Whitehouse Station (NJ): Merck Research Laboratories; 2006. p. 85–9.
2. Walton J, Tarondess JA, Lock S, editors. The oxford medical companion. Oxford: Oxford University Press; 1994. p. 154, 236.
3. McLemore LJ. Inflammatory bowel disease. Radiol Technol 2007;78(4):291–309.
4. Coleman J. Patient assessment: gastrointestinal system. In: Morton PG, Fontaine DK, Hudak CM, et al, editors. Critical care nursing: a holistic approach. Philadelphia: Lippincott Williams & Wilkins; 2005. p. 911–31.
5. American Gastroenterological Association. AGA patient center page. Available at: http://www.gastro.org/wmspage.cfm?parm1=860. Accessed May 28, 2009.
6. Loperfido S, Caroli A. Post-ERCP perforation. UpToDate 2009. Available at: http://www.uptodate.com/online/content/topic.do?topicKey=biliaryt/11761&view=print. Accessed April 23, 2009.
7. Mallery JS, Baron TH, Dominitz JA, et al. Complications of ERCP. Gastrointest Endosc 2003;57(6):633–8. Available from: American Society for Gastrointestinal Endoscopy. Available at: http://www.sciencedirect.com.proxy.library.vanderbilt.edu/science?_ob=MImg&_imagekey=B6WFY-4C1DRYV-2-1&_cdi=6807&_user=86629&_orig=browse&_coverDate=05%2F31%2F2003&_sk=999429993&view=c&wchp=dGLbV1b-zSkWb&md5=de20d13a04a48060122bf8c9eafca8d7&ie=/sdarticle.pdf. Accessed May 13, 2009.
8. Trap R, Adamsen S, Hart-Hansen O, et al. Severe and fatal complications after diagnostic and therapeutic ERCP: a prospective series of claims to insurance covering public hospitals. Endoscopy 1999;31(2):125–30.
9. Choi CW, Kang DH, Kim GH, et al. Nafamostat mesylate in the prevention of post-ERCP pancreatitis and risk factors for post-ERCP pancreatitis. Gastrointest Endosc 2009;69(4):e12–8.
10. Shojamanesh H, Roy PK, Nwakakwa V. Cholangitis. eMedicine [serial online]. June 2006. Available at: http://emedicine.medscape.com/article/184043-overview. Accessed May 13, 2009.
11. Gladden D, Migala AF, Beverly CS, et al. Cholecystitis. eMedicine [serial online]. August 2008. Available at: http://emedicine.medscape.com/article/171886-overview. Accessed May 13, 2009.
12. Cariani G, Di Marco M, Roda E, et al. Efficacy and safety of ERCP in patients 90 years of age and older. Gastrointest Endosc 2006;64(3):471–2.
13. Yusuf TE, Wofford SA, Bhutani MS. Esophagogastroduodenoscopy. eMedicine [serial online]. August 2007. Available at: http://emedicine.medscape.com/article/185016-overview. Accessed May 13, 2009.
14. Allen K, Berry DM, Blumenthal NP, et al. Portable diagnostic tests. Philadelphia: Lippincott Williams & Wilkins; 2007. Available at: http://booksgoogle.com/books?id=QA1LdHAuE7kC&pg=PA134&lpg=PA134&dq=nursing+implications+capsule+endoscopy&source=bl&ots=i4PJmIqe_H&sig=He20hyvRr2M_K3e-NF68yzdRdd4&hl=en&ei=K-BSvv6AoTQMrKQvd0H&sa=X&oi=book_result&ct=result&resnum=8#PPA134, M1. Accessed May 28, 2009.

15. Marks JW. Capsule endoscopy (wireless capsule endoscopy). Medicinenet.com [serial online]. 2009. Available at: http://www.medicinenet.com/capsule_endo scopy/article.htm. Accessed May 13, 2000.

16. American Society of Gastrointestinal Endoscopy. Understanding UES (endo-scopic ultrasonography). Available at: http://www.asge.org/PatientInfoIndex. aspx?id=380. Accessed May 13, 2009.

17. Mayo Clinic. Endoscopic ultrasound page. Available at: http://www.mayoclinic. org/endoscopic-ultrasound/. Accessed May 28, 2009.

18. Kita H. Overview of double balloon endoscopy. UptoDate; 2009. Available at: http://www.uptodate.com/online/content/topic.do?topicKey=gi_endos/11935&view =print. Accessed April 23, 2009.

19. Lichtenstein G. Bowel preparations for colonoscopy: a review. Am J Health Syst Pharm 2009;66(1):27–37.

20. Taber's cyclopedic medical dictionary, 1989.

21. A-Rahim YI, Falchuk M. Bowel preparation for colonoscopy. UptoDate; 2009. Available at: http://www.uptodate.com/online/content/topic.do?topicKey=gi_ endos/6324&view=print. Accessed April 23, 2009.

22. Charette A. Patient information: colonoscopy. UpToDate; 2009. Available at: http://www.uptodate.com/online/content/topic.do?topicKey=digestiv/5496&view =print. Accessed April 23, 2009.

23. Christ AD, Bauerfeind P, Gyr N. Peritonitis after colonoscopy in a patient with ascites. Endoscopy 1993;25:553–4.

24. Quallick MR, Brown WR. Rectal perforation during colonoscopic retroflexion: a large prospective experience in an academic center. Gastrointest Endosc. 2009;69(4):960–3.

25. Vellacott KD. Septicemia after colonoscopy due to an Iliac artery aneurysm. Endoscopy 1984;16:35.

26. Baumann UA, Mettler M. Diagnosis and hazards of unexpected diaphragmatic hernias during colonoscopy: report of two cases. Endoscopy 1999;31(3):274–6.

27. Ylinen E, Vehvilainen-Julkunen K, Pietila A. Nurses' knowledge and skills in colo-noscopy patients' pain management. J Clin Nurs 2007;16:1125–33.

28. Charette A. Patient information: flexible sigmoidoscopy. UpToDate; 2009. Available at: http://www.uptodate.com/online/content/topic.do?topicKey=digestiv/6940&view =print. Accessed April 23, 2009.

29. WebMD, 2007. Available at: http://www.webmd.com/digestive-disorders/sigmoid oscopy-anoscopy-proctoscopy. Accessed May 13, 2009.

30. Lazzaroni M, Porro GB. Preparation, premedication, and surveillance. Endoscopy 2001;33(2):103–8.

Bronchoscopy: What Critical Care Nurses Need to Know

Dixie L. Taylor, BSN, RN

KEYWORDS

- Bronchoscopy • Moderate sedation • Specimen
- Tracheal intubations • Patient education • Pneumothorax

Critical care nurses encounter patients undergoing bronchoscope studies in the outpatient setting, inpatient setting, and sometimes even at the bedside. The bronchoscope has an important role as a diagnostic tool in the fields of thoracic surgery and internal medicine. This tool, commonly used today, has a rich history. The first bronchoscopy was performed by Gustav Killian in 1897.[1–3] Over the last one hundred years, the bronchoscope has evolved from a conventional rigid scope, to a fiberscope, to the now commonly used combination of the fiberscope and video-assisted rigid and flexible fiberscope. The flexible fiberoptic broncho-scope (FFB) was developed in 1964 by Ikeda, and has led to a clinical science of bronchoscopy.[3] Approximately 500,000 bronchoscopic procedures are done annually in the United States.[4,5]

THE FFB EXAMINATION

During the FFB examination, a fiberoptic tube composed of a light and mirrors is used to visualize the airway while oxygen is administered via the tube. The bronchoscope may be inserted oropharyngeally or nasopharyngeally. Bronchoscopy may be used emergently, as in the removal of a foreign body, or as an elective procedure and can serve either diagnostic or therapeutic purposes. Because of the potential for severe, although rare, adverse events during the procedure, FFB should always be performed by an experienced physician. It is usually performed by a surgeon or a pulmonologist, and takes from 30 minutes to an hour. FFB can be performed at the bedside, an operating room, or an endoscopy suite. It can be done on an outpatient or inpatient basis.

Department of Medical Intensive Care, Vanderbilt University Medical Center, 1211 Medical Drive, Nashville, TN 37232, USA
E-mail address: dixie.taylor@vanderbilt.edu

Crit Care Nurs Clin N Am 22 (2010) 33–40
doi:10.1016/j.ccell.2009.10.004
0899-5885/10/$ – see front matter
ccnursing.theclinics.com

COMMON INDICATIONS

There is a wide range of diagnostic and therapeutic indications for bronchoscopy. The usual indications for a bronchoscope are diagnostic, with the most common patient being someone who has presented with clinical or radiologic suspicions of cancer.[6] Other common indications include evaluation of hemoptysis and further possible biopsy of abnormal growths found during radiology studies. Sputum or washings of cells for cytology studies may be collected for diagnostic purposes. Grading and staging of neoplasms can be performed when the bronchoscope includes a biopsy.[6] **Table 1** provides an overview of the main diagnostic and therapeutic indications for a bronchoscopy. Additionally, difficult intubations are performed via bronchoscopy so that the patient may undergo less trauma than that experienced with multiple unsuccessful attempts. A physician may wish to observe the respiratory system of a patient who has had recurrent issues with unexplained pneumothorax. Pneumonia may indicate the need for a bronchial examination (washing may be sent to the lab for identification of the growth). Abnormal breathing may indicate the need for further examination. The removal of mucous plugs can successfully be removed via a bronchoscope. As with all invasive procedures, bronchoscopy should only be performed with patient consent.

CONTRAINDICATIONS

Absolute contraindications include inability to keep the patient oxygenated during the procedure and hemodynamic instability. Relative contraindications include elevated prothrombin time or international normalized ratio, low platelet count, chronic obstructive pulmonary disease, asthma, or recent myocardial infarction. The procedure may need to be aborted if the patient becomes hypoxic, hypercarbic, or bradycardic. There has been much discussion about the feasibility and safety of the procedure for

Table 1
Age specific considerations

Pediatric	Geriatric
The most common indication for bronchoscopy for children is for the removal of a foreign body from the larynx or trachea	Higher risk for hypothermia. Monitor temperature and provide warm blankets
A laryngeal mask airway is often used to stabilize the airway	Observe for signs and symptoms of dehydration, as patient has been NPO
Higher risk of hypoxemia because their airways are smaller and more fragile	Restlessness can be an indication of hypoxemia; monitor oxygen saturations closely
Obtain a baseline of the patient's level of communication skills. For patients who do not communicate appropriately, observe more closely regarding temperature, hypoxemia, and pain	Obtain a baseline of the patient's level of communication skills. For patients who do not communicate appropriately observe more closely, regarding temperature, hypoxemia, and pain
Postprocedure care includes physiotherapy (as needed), monitoring vital signs, and caregiver education	May be more likely to experience postprocedure pain related to positioning
Review medications held due to NPO status and administer as directed	Review medications held due to NPO status and administer as directed

patients with pulmonary hypertension; however, there is now evidence to support that FFB can be done safely in patients with mild-to-moderate pulmonary hypertension.[7]

COMPLICATIONS

FBB has been performed for over 35 years and is considered a very safe procedure with low rates of morbidity and mortality.[8] Serious risks, such as air leak or serious bleeding, occur less than 5% of the time.[9] There are a variety of complications that can and do occur during a bronchoscopy.[8–14] The more common complications and explanations are offered in **Table 2**.

SEDATION DURING BRONCHOSCOPY

There continues to be a great deal of discussion about which medications, if any, should be used during a bronchoscopy. This is contingent upon the preference of the person doing the test and there is a wide variance in current practice. Some diagnosticians prefer not to sedate the patient at all during this procedure. The thought behind this is that half of the major complications related to the procedure are related to the sedation and not the mechanics of the procedure itself. In general, some form of sedation is used to alleviate fear and anxiety, and to promote patient comfort. If the procedure is not painful or unpleasant, the likelihood of a patient consenting to additional testing increases.

There have been numerous studies about the efficacy and effects of different agents used during bronchoscopic procedures to alleviate pain, cough, dyspnea, and anxiety.[15] A variety of medications have been used over the years, the most common being benzodiazepines, opioids, and, to a lesser, extent propofol.[15] A drug that is currently being studied for its efficacy during bronchoscopic procedures is fospropofol disodium.[16] This is the first new drug in 19 years to be studied for this purpose. It is a water soluble prodrug of propofol with pharmacokinetic and pharmacodynamic properties that are not the same as propofol emulsion. Fospropofol appears to hold much promise as a sedative during bronchoscopy. The drug has a rapid recovery, a favorable safety profile, and warrants more study for consideration as a drug of choice for bronchoscopic procedures.[15–17]

MONITORING AND PATIENT SAFETY

Institutions where bronchoscopies are performed should have institutional guidelines for sedation and analgesia. Continuous monitoring of pulse oximetry, electrocardiography, respiratory rate, and blood pressure are common for bronchoscopic procedures. To reduce the risk of aspiration, the patient should not have anything orally for at least 6 hours before the procedure.[8] Equipment for advanced airway management, and suctioning should be immediately available, along with a cardiac defibrillator and advanced life support medications.

STAFF SAFETY

All personnel involved in the procedure should practice universal safety precautions. It is important to have knowledge of the patient's history and physical status to know if precautions that are more stringent are advised. The patient may require or be on respiratory isolation. In situations where tuberculosis a consideration, the appropriate N95 masks should be worn by the staff. Additionally, it is recommended that staff be vaccinated against hepatitis B and titer levels should be confirmed. During the procedure, staff should wear protective equipment including gowns, masks or visors, and

Table 2
Common complications related to bronchoscopic procedures

Complication	Discussion
Discomfort and coughing	The bronchoscope may cause some pain, discomfort and coughing while passing through the airway. The local analgesic will reduce the gag reflex and reduce the pain induced by the scope. Medication given intravenously will reduce sensation
Hypoxemia	Hypoxemia can occur during any phase of the procedure. Hypoxemia can occur in cases where the bronchoscope blocks airflow into the lungs or in cases where over-sedation results in alveolar collapse. Oxygen is administered during the procedure. Oxygen saturations should be monitored throughout the procedure with the goal of keeping saturations above or at 90%. If oxygen saturations stay low, the procedure may be aborted
Hypotension	A dehydrated patient is particularly susceptible to hypotension. Fluids or medications may be administered depending on the severity and cause of the hypotension
Cardiac arrhythmias and ischemia	Significant hemodynamic alterations occur during bronchoscopy. Mean arterial pressure, heart rate, and cardiac index increase as the scope passes through the larynx and during suctioning. The incidence of arrhythmias during the procedure is variable and can include tachycardia, premature atrial and ventricular contractions, atrial fibrillation, atrial flutter, bradycardia, supraventricular tachycardia, and ventricular tachycardia
Laryngospasm	Stimulation by the scope may induce laryngospasm in some patients
Pneumothorax	A pneumothorax is more likely to occur when a biopsy is taken, although this complication is uncommon. The staff needs to be prepared to insert a chest tube when indicated. The incidence of pneumothorax in patients undergoing biopsy is reported to be between 5% and 11.8%. A chest radiograph about 1 hour after bronchoscopy is recommended to exclude the presence of a pneumothorax

Bleeding	Bleeding can occur after the physician performs a biopsy or if the bronchoscope injures the airway or a tumor within the airway. Bleeding is more likely to occur if the airway is already diseased. Medication can be administered through the bronchoscope to stop bleeding if necessary. Before this procedure, it is important to know the patient's international normalized ratio level and any risk factors such as immunosuppressed status, thrombocytopenia, uremia, liver disease, coagulopathies, and severe pulmonary hypertension
Fever	Fever following flexible bronchoscopy is reported to occur in about 5%–30% of the cases. The fever usually is brief and subsides within 24 hours. Fever appears to be related to the release of proinflammatory cytokines that are stimulated during the procedure
Pneumonia	The incidence of pneumonia occurs in about 6% of bronchoscopy cases. Infrequently, bacteremia following bronchoscopy has been reported
Adverse drug reaction	The nurse needs to be alert for drug reactions, as this may occur as the result of medications given before and during the procedure

gloves. Sharps should not be resheathed. Equipment should be cleaned according to policy and, whenever possible, disposable accessories should be used.

PREPARING THE PATIENT FOR THE PROCEDURE

Although institutional guidelines about the specifics of preparing the patient may vary, **Box 1** explains common considerations that warrant use across settings and institutions.

POSTPROCEDURE CONSIDERATIONS

When the procedure is over, there are certain guidelines that should be used to insure patient safety and to minimize postprocedure complications. As with all clients who have received tracheal-bronchial anesthesia, do not allow client to eat or drink until the anesthesia has worn off and the gag reflex has returned. Be sure to remove the patient's intravenous access before discharge, and make certain the patient has transportation home and is given written discharge instructions. Make certain the bronchoscope is sent for proper sterilization as provided by the institution's policy.

DISCHARGE TEACHING

There are several common points that should be covered thoroughly when discharging a client after bronchoscopy. Clients should be instructed to notify the provider of the following symptoms: fever, chest pain, dyspnea, wheezing, or hemoptysis (patients should be instructed to report more than few tablespoons of blood, a small amount is to be expected—especially when a biopsy has been performed). Patients should not eat or drink until the numbness of the throat has worn off, usually half an hour to an hour. Patients and family or caregivers should be given contact information in the event of complications. Patients should understand that throat discomfort is normal and that they may use throat lozenges or throat spray for relief of symptoms.

Box 1
Patient preparation for the bronchoscopy

Identify the client using two identifiers—consult the institution's policy

Verify patient has patent intravenous access, which is necessary throughout the procedure for administering sedation. Intravenous access should remain patent until the patient is recovered

Verify dentures have been removed, when applicable

Verify that informed consent has been obtained

Obtain vital signs and oxygen saturation

Assess respiratory status, including type of cough, sputum production, and lung sound

Determine purpose of procedure

Determine client's allergies; make certain that no anesthetics planned for use are contraindicated

Assess need for preprocedure medication, such as atropine

Assess time client last ingested food. Make sure this is congruent to the institutional policy

Assess client's level of understanding of the procedure including any fears, concerns, and anxieties

All discharge instructions should be reinforced by written instructions given to the patient or caregiver at the time of discharge.

Arrangement should be made for follow-up appointments. It is also important to communicate clearly about procedures and proper expectations for feedback from any pending test. The physician can give the laboratory results to the patient while inspecting the lung before discharge. Specimens sent to the lab for testing could take several days for interpretation. Instruct the patient on when results should be expected and how this will be communicated to the patient or family. Also, instruct them on how to follow-up should they not hear from the physician's office within the anticipated time-frame.

COMMUNICATION

Communication is essential in providing excellent patient care. Effective communication between the members of the medical team and between the physician and the patient, family, or caregiver is imperative. Common fears of patients include pain, breathing difficulties, oropharyngeal irritation, bronchoscopy findings and their implications, sedation, and cross-infection. Physicians are more likely to explain the indications for a bronchoscopy than the actual procedure and what the patient can anticipate postprocedure.[18] Medical personnel can assist in alleviating fear by offering education in the physician's office once the patient realizes the need for a bronchoscopy. The medical staff can explain the preprocedure expectations, the procedure itself, and the postprocedure expectations. With increased anxiety, the patient may need to have information repeated to process the information. If possible, have a family member, significant other, or caregiver present during the teaching times. Let the patient know he or she will need someone to transport him or her home if this is an outpatient procedure.

Shortly before the procedure, remind the patient what to expect while the bronchoscopy is being performed. Explain the need for an intravenous line, the laryngeal sedation, the use of moderate sedation, the scope, the monitors and their purposes, the loss of gag reflex, and the need to expectorate the local anesthetic. Explain the indications, the suction, and sounds associated with the suction. If the patient remains conscious during the procedure, provide explanations as to what is occurring and what to expect next. For example, "The physician is now viewing the larynx. The procedure is going well. We have approximately 3 minutes left."

SUMMARY

Bronchoscopic procedures have been performed for over one hundred years. They are relatively safe when practice guidelines are followed. However, they are invasive and a real source of anxiety and fear for the patient. Although there are complications that can and do occur during a bronchoscopy, being attuned to the potential complications and knowing appropriate interventions will ameliorate the consequences of these obstacles and effect best patient outcomes. The role of the nurse is essential—from the initial teaching about the procedure to the discharge of the patient.

REFERENCES

1. Zhang J, Wang CL. The history of the evolvement of bronchoscope. Zhonghua Yi Shi Za Zhi 2006;36(2):96–9.
2. Prakesh UBS. Gustav Killian centenary: the celebration of a century of progress in bronchoscopy. J Bronchol 1997;4:1–2.

3. Ouelette DR. The safety of bronchoscopy in a fellowship program. Chest 2006; 130:1185–90.

4. Kirschke DL, Jones TF, Craig AS, et al. *Pseudomonas aeruginosa* and *Serratia marcescens* contamination associated with a manufacturing defect in bronchoscopes. N Engl J Med 2003;348(3):214–20.

5. DePriest K, Wahla A, Chatterjee A, et al. Bronchoscopic myths and legends: bronchoscopy and endocarditis prophylaxis. Clin Pulm Med 2009;16:51–3.

6. Postmus P. Bronchoscopy for lung cancer. Chest 2005;128:16–8.

7. Diaz-Guzman E, Vadi S, Minai OA, et al. Safety of diagnostic bronchoscopy in patients with pulmonary hypertension. Respiration 2009;77:292–7.

8. Gorman SR, Beamis JF. Complications of flexible bronchoscopy. Clin Pulm Med 2005;12:177–83.

9. Patient information series: fiberoptic bronchoscopy. American Thoracic Society. Available at: www.thoracic.org. Accessed November 1, 2009.

10. Um S, Choi C, Lee C, et al. Prospective analysis of clinical characteristics and risk factors of postbronchoscopy fever. Chest 2004;125:945–52.

11. Watanabe A, Saka H, Shimokata K, et al. Fever and bacteremia following flexible bronchoscopy. J Bronchol 1994;1:5–8.

12. Pereira W, Kovnat DM, Khan MA, et al. Fever and pneumonia after flexible fiberoptic bronchoscopy. Am Rev Respir Dis 1975;112:59–64.

13. Witte MC, Opal SM, Gilbert JG, et al. Incidence of fever and bacteremia following transbronchial needle aspiration. Chest 1986;89:85–7.

14. Krause A, Hohberg B, Heine F, et al. Cytokines derived from alveolar macrophages induce fever after bronchoscopy and bronchoalveolar lavage. Am J Respir Crit Care Med 1997;155:1793–7.

15. Jantz MA. The old and new of sedation for bronchoscopy. Chest 2009;135:4–6.

16. Silvestri GA, Vincent BD, Wahidi MM, et al. A phase 3, randomized, double-blind, study to assess the efficacy and safety of fospropofol disodium injection for moderate sedation in patients undergoing flexible bronchoscopy. Chest 2009; 135:41–7.

17. Cohen LB. Clinical trial: a dose-response study of fospropofol disodium for moderate sedation during colonoscopy. Aliment Pharmacol Ther 2008;27: 597–608.

18. Poi PJH, Chuah SY, Srinivas P, et al. Common fears of patients undergoing bronchoscopy. Eur Respir J 1998;6(2):133–4.

Radiographic Studies in the Critical Care Environment

Maria A. Revell, DSN, RN, COI[a],*, Marcia Pugh, MSN, MBA, HCM[b],
Tasha L. Smith, BS[c], Leigh Ann McInnis, PhD, RN, FNP-BC[a]

KEYWORDS

- Critical care • Computed tomography • Radiography
- Radiographic imaging • Magnetic resonance imaging

Critical care patients present with or develop conditions that require imaging with a variety of radiographic methods, which give health care providers quick access to internal body information for rapid interpretation and patient management. These methods provide a wealth of detailed information in a short period of time for the health care provider. Most noninvasive radiographic techniques are relatively quick and safe, with low complication rates. Technological advances such as the introduction of digital imaging instead of screen-film radiography have improved image resolution, readability, management, and portability of results while maintaining confidentiality of patient information. These methods promote increased use of radiography as a standard method of patient management that the critical care nurse must be cognizant of in this high-acuity setting.

Radiographic procedures are an integral part of patient management, and require an elevated level of understanding by the critical care nurse. This process goes beyond merely glancing at radiographs for self awareness but involves viewing the radiographic study as an integral part of the pathway for managing complex patient situations. Radiographic enhancements have given critical care nurses "point and click" bedside access to patient imaging results. Computer-generated high-quality diagnostic images are available quickly when required, and give a patient view that facilitates emergent management.

Bedside radiographic procedures are becoming commonplace occurrences. Technological innovations have made this tool one that can significantly enhance clinical

[a] School of Nursing, Middle Tennessee State University, PO Box 81, Murfreesboro, TN 37132, USA
[b] Grants, Research and Outreach of West AL Division, Tombigbee Healthcare Authority, PO Box 890, Demopolis, AL 36732, USA
[c] Cardiac Management, Medtronic, 8200 Coral Sea North East, MVC23, Mounds View, MN 55112, USA
* Corresponding author.
E-mail address: massmith@mtsu.edu (M.A. Revell).

Crit Care Nurs Clin N Am 22 (2010) 41–50
doi:10.1016/j.ccell.2009.10.013
0899-5885/10/$ – see front matter © 2010 Elsevier Inc. All rights reserved.

management. Radiographic procedures can be easily performed, and the results are readily and quickly available. The use of these procedures has enabled care providers to offer efficient, cost-effective critical care. Radiographic procedures can be a catalyst in the collaborative management format of care, and promote optimized real-time care management techniques.

Radiographic imaging techniques can be performed for various body parts and for any number of reasons, for example, diagnostic or interventional purpose. Diagnostic radiology includes radiographic imaging of specific body parts, catheter angiography, computed tomography (CT), and magnetic resonance imaging (MRI). Interventional radiology includes arterial/venous interventions and vascular access procedures.

Daily chest radiographs historically were performed for all patients in the critical care setting. These procedures were often done due to patient placement (ie, critical care setting), not because of any specific patient condition. The clinical value of this technique has been questioned. Research has validated that the prediction of changes in patient conditions was extremely low.[1] Studies also validated that daily chest radiographs seldom prompted action, as they did not reveal clinically relevant abnormalities.[1,2] Research demonstrated that the diagnostic yield for this intervention in a mixed medical-surgical intensive care unit was relatively low, although this may differ for other types of intensive care units. Based on this research and others undertaken over the past 10 years, many institutions have excluded routine daily chest radiographs in critical care settings.[1,3–5] Despite ambivalence related to chest radiographs, this is an important procedure that yields rapid and efficient information for intervention when indicated.

Radiographs of other body parts can also be used to validate suspected changes for intervention. Although often done for evaluation of skeletal alterations, the routine radiograph can give information related to body organs. Diagnostic evaluation of diseases that affect soft tissue can also be accomplished through a routine radiograph. Bedside radiographic procedures may not give specific details, but they can be used for identification of localized areas requiring further evaluation by CT or MRI. Diagnostic imaging gives specific information regarding size, position, and anatomic alteration of emergent conditions such as pneumothorax, hemithorax, and effusions.

SPECIFIC RADIOGRAPHIC EVALUATION

Radiographic evaluation includes chest radiographs, CT of various body parts, and MRI evaluation. Areas commonly diagnostically imaged include the head, chest, abdomen, and pelvis. These areas can be evaluated using the range of radiographic studies from simple bedside radiography to complex MRI evaluation.

BEDSIDE ANTEROPOSTERIOR RADIOGRAPHY

Obtaining radiographic imaging at the bedside allows patient management of the patient in the critical care setting without the potential for additional complications related to transport. Bedside anteroposterior chest radiography is one of the most common critical care radiographic procedures. What it lacks in sensitivity when compared with the CT scan, it makes up for in ease and speed of results retrieval. This anteroposterior procedure is one of the first radiographic methods used for patients who have emergent situations that require internal views of the chest and abdomen. This radiological format is useful for evaluation of critically ill patients and those who have undergone surgical intervention.[6] Among conditions that may warrant bedside evaluation are (to name a few) suspected pneumothorax; hemothorax; congestive heart failure; effusions of the heart and lungs; pulmonary edema[7]; kidney, ureter, and bladder abnormalities; and abdominal masses.

Reviewing radiographic results is a skill. However, there are standard points that can be used by the critical care nurse to recognize and distinguish normal anatomic structures. Developing the ability to distinguish these structures allows the nurse to identify gross abnormalities that warrant notification of other collaborative health care members.

Anteroposterior chest radiographs are the most frequent radiographic tests performed in the critical care setting. Gross review by the critical care nurse can reveal a wealth of information that can be used for quick patient intervention in emergent situations. Quick review should never be used as the sole determinant for intervention. Nursing assessment findings are key indicators of required interventions. When reviewing a film, the nurse should verify left to right and top to bottom image placement, then move from identification of tubes and lines to soft tissue and bones (**Table 1**).[8,9] This brief outline will not create an expert radiological reader, but is intended to give

Table 1
Chest radiographic structure identification

Area	Radiographic Structure	Visually Normal Findings
Chest/abdomen	Endotracheal tube, nasogastric/orogastric tube, hemodynamic monitoring catheter, cardiac pacemaker/ defibrillator	Device outline and markings should be apparent on visualization
Soft tissue	Neck, supraclavicular, axilla, chest wall, breast, abdomen, gastric bubble	Supraclavicular, axillary, breast, and lateral soft tissue silhouette
Bones	Humerus, shoulder joint, scapula, clavicle, vetebrae, ribs, sternum	The number of ribs should be obtainable from an actual count. Structures are clearly visible and articulations present
Heart and mediastinum	Heart, major vessels, mediastinum	Heart shadow should be less than half the width of the thoracic cage. Inferior vena cava, cardiac borders, aortic arch, and descending aorta should be visible
Upper abdomen	Diaphragm, abdominal organs, gastric bubble	Liver and spleen should be identifiable. Costophrenic angles should be sharp and well defined.[9] The gas-filled stomach should be visible below the diaphragm
Lungs	Trachea, bronchial structure, hilum, vasculature, apices.	Tracheal air column, carina, and linear and fine nodular shadows of pulmonary vessels can be seen

a better understanding of areas for review for patient management and more effective health care team collaboration.

When reviewing these anatomic areas, structures of increased density will appear white (eg, bony structures) while areas with less density will appear dark (eg, air filled lungs, gastric air bubble). Body organs will take on various appearances based on their density (eg, heart, liver, areas of varied consolidation) (**Fig. 1**).

This form of assessment is not without its pitfalls. If the patient has a poor inspiratory effort or the film is taken on ventilatory expiration, structures will appear crowded in the thoracic cavity due to the height of the diaphragm. Lung markings will not be clear and the cardiac margins may be obscured. If adequate penetration of the film is not achieved, results may be exaggerated or obliterated. The test of a good film is when the thoracic rib markings can be visualized over the cardiac silhouette. It is also important for the patient to be perpendicular to the film. Lateral rotation can result in unequal clavicular distances. This mechanism is one that can be used for verification of proper positioning. It is important that critical care nurses facilitate proper patient positioning to obtain the best anteroposterior radiograph possible.

COMPUTED TOMOGRAPHY

CT, previously called computed axial tomography (CAT), historically derived from a form of geometric image processing that developed a 3-dimensional image from multiple 2-dimensional ones taken from an axial view. The clinical inception of this was in the 1970s. CT has proved to be an evolution of medicine that promotes innovative advances that continue today.[10] The term CAT has not been used for several years, simply leaving the term CT scan.

CT produces a series of attenuation (density) profiles from narrowly collimated x-ray beams. These beams pass through the body at various angles, which produces a series of attenuation profiles. This information is then computer-processed to generate an image using various shades of gray. Based on density, body tissues attenuate the x-ray beam at different rates. The resulting image allows for determination of various components: fatty, cystic, or mineralized.[11]

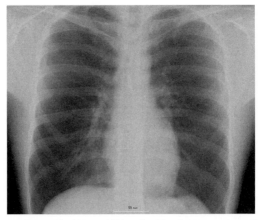

Fig. 1. Normal chest radiograph. (*From* Wikipedia: The free encyclopedia. Wikimedia Foundation. Available at: http://commons.wikimedia.org/wiki/File:Chest.png. This image is licensed under the GNU Free Documentation License.)

CT scans have become an indisputable adjunct to radiographic and ultrasonic images in the critical care setting. CT scanning is used in a large number of abnormality verification and identification for multiple body parts. Due to procedure cost, it is not often used for initial defect identification. The CT scanning mechanism gives health care providers the option to visualize structures with or without the use of contrast (**Fig. 2**), allowing for scanning of thin sections with high spatial frequency reconstructions. This latter form of CT scanning is called high-resolution computed tomography (HRCT). HRCT often does not result in a full graphical depiction of body structures, but is used for intense evaluation of selected portions of body structures.

The majority of graphical images viewed by health care providers will be 2-dimensional. The CT scanner can actually retrieve a graphic 3-dimensional image even though the operator visualizes a 2-dimensional one (see **Fig. 2**). The CT scanner can render a 3-dimensional image for visualization if the scanner is equipped with special computer software, resulting in a 3-dimensional representation of the body structure.

CT has improved lesion characterization over standard radiography. CT gives more defined characterization to soft tissue and bony formations, and allows for clear identification of abnormalities where anatomic configuration is more complex (eg, spine and pelvis). Not only does it give refined delineation to normal bony structures, but the architecture of bony lesions is also easily identified. The CT scan has the ability to depict subtle differences in tissue density, which makes it a very good diagnostic tool for not only identifying abnormalities but also for delineating tissue type and tumor involvement.[11]

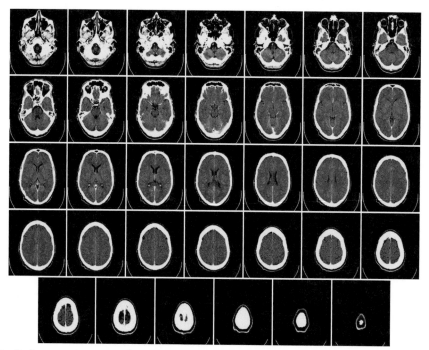

Fig. 2. Computed tomography with contrast of brain from skull to top of skull. (*From* Wikipedia: The free encyclopedia. Wikimedia Foundation. Available at: http://commons.wikimedia. org/wiki/File:Chest.png. This image is licensed under the GNU Free Documentation License.)

VOLUME COMPUTED TOMOGRAPHY

Volume computed tomography (VCT) is the newest innovation in patient imaging. The Lightspeed VCT was brought to the forefront of medical imaging in 2004. This device is able to capture any organ in 1 second. VCT can perform a total body scan in less than 10 seconds. This scanner allows retrieval of conditions of blood vessels in key body organs such as the heart and brain. Within 5 cardiac beats the scanner can retrieve submillimeter resolution high-quality images of the coronary architecture. VCT can give access to brain circulatory components in reduced time, to allow for quick initiation of stroke treatment and intervention for myocardial infarctions.[12] This technology allows access to more 3-dimensional scanning technology and thus more thorough surface assessment of bony structures, permitting a full view from all directions.[13]

MAGNETIC RESONANCE IMAGING

MRI technology is relatively new when compared with basic radiography. This technology was introduced in 1973 whereas radiographic images of the body have been in existence since 1895. The knowledge gained in the study of nuclear MRI led to the development of this radiographic technique for use in health care.[14]

MRI is a complex process that uses the signal from the nuclei of hydrogen atoms to generate an image. The positively charged single proton of the hydrogen atom has a negatively charged electron that rotates around it. The proton possesses spin, which means that it rotates around its axis. Because the proton rotates with an electrical charge, it has magnetic moment and acts like a small magnet. Protons normally rotate in random directions. The external magnet causes the protons to line up parallel to the main magnetic field. After these are aligned a radiofrequency pulse generates an MR signal. The banging sound heard during MRI is the radio pulse or waves, rapidly switching on and off. Radiofrequency waves cause the protons that are lined up with the magnetic field to flip 90°. Protons will go back to their original position whenever the radio pulse switches off, which causes them to emit an electromagnetic signal. This signal is collected and processed by the computer to generate an image.[10,15]

MRI scanners have great technical flexibility. The scanner can be specifically calibrated to highlight specific tissue types. Fatty tissue is best imaged with a T1-weighted imaging sequence, whereas fluids are best imaged with a T2-weighted sequence. These techniques can be combined with 3-dimensional MRI to identify tumor shape and size. The use of contrast agents can further facilitate delineation of abnormality specifics.

An MRI scan can produce detailed soft tissue and organ information. MRI scans can be used intraoperatively to pinpoint tumors for precision during surgical intervention in a lead-shielded surgical suite.[15,16] This situation allows for the detection of small structural changes, especially when gadolinium is used as a contrast agent. Because the machine has a strong magnet, it is imperative to identify if the patient harbors any metallic structures. For individuals who work in metal machine shops or weld metal objects for a profession, this usually means obtaining a preliminary head radiograph to identify metallic objects that may be lodged in the eyes. It is important to obtain a history of any object that could possibly contain metal as a component, such as intrauterine devices, cochlear implants, pacemakers or pacemaker/defibrillators, brain aneurysm clips, and so forth. Historical information should also include conditions such as claustrophobia, which can result in an inability to initiate or complete the scan without administration of antianxiety medication.

CT AND MRI: UNDERSTANDING THE DIFFERENCE

Both CT and MRI have made dramatic impacts in radiographic evaluation for patients in the critical care setting. CT scans result in geometrically precise scans; however, they give less soft tissue information. MRI quality exceeds CT in this area. CT generates less movement artifact but can result in bone artifact. MRI image quality exceeds CT in evaluation of bones of the head. With contrast use, CT scans are better for detecting meningiomas of the head. MRI has proved to be more specific in identification of tumor volume, and can lead to more defined treatment modalities for addressing cranial tumors.[17] MRI was also found to be more sensitive than CT in detecting brain metastasis during preoperative evaluation of patients with potentially operable cancer of the lung.[18] In pleural disease, CT scans are sensitive for calcification detection. The sensitivity and specificity of MRI in the detection of pleural malignancy exceeds that of CT imaging.[19] It is not uncommon to see CT and MRI used concurrently to retrieve complementary information from both scanning techniques (**Table 2**). This dual use gives the health care team the best information possible to make decisions regarding health care modalities to be used for the best patient outcome.

Table 2
CT and MRI comparisons

	CT	MRI
Image creation	Uses ionizing radiation	Uses magnet and nonionizing radiofrequency signals
Patient positioning	Machine rotates around patient	Patient placed in magnetic machine
Machine dynamics	Relatively noise free	Machine is noisy and patient must remain perfectly still
Soft tissue resolution	Less detailed than with MRI	Good detail
Bony resolution	Good detail	Less detailed than with CT
Imaging plane	Older machines cannot produce images in any plane. Multidetector scanners can produce images in any plane	Can produce images in any plane without moving the patient
Contrast media	Iodine-based contrast are absorbed by abnormal tissues.	Noniodine-based with fewer documented cases of reactions
Contrast images	Cannot change the contrast of images	Can change the contrast of the images through small changes in the radio waves and the magnetic fields. Different contrast settings will highlight different types of tissue
Contraindications to use	Patients for whom radiation exposure is contraindicated such as pregnancy; multiple tests required over short period of time	Patients with metal in their body and devices such as pacemakers cannot be tested in this manner

ROLE OF THE CRITICAL CARE NURSE

The role of the critical care nurse in radiographic imaging is based on the radiographic study performed. It is important to be familiar with the organization's policies and procedures related to patient management and performance of procedures. The nurse needs to know any special preparation required for radiographic procedures. Failure to adequately prepare the patient may result in delay or cancellation of the procedure. For the patient in the critical care unit, this may cause significant delays in medical treatment or surgical intervention that rely on procedure results.

Written or electronic request for the procedure should be clear and succinct. Any special consent forms required must be obtained before narcotic or mind-altering

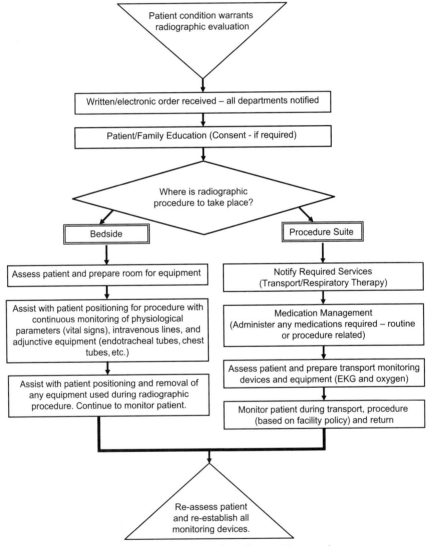

Fig. 3. Flow diagram of patient management in radiographic procedures.

drug administration. The family should be given instructions regarding the procedure, waiting areas, and when procedures are to be done. Whether the study is performed at the bedside or in the procedure suite, patient education is imperative. Instructions should be given in terms the patient and family can understand. Studies that can be performed at the bedside require that the nurse be especially attentive to changes in the patient's condition during all phases of the procedure (**Fig. 3**).

SUMMARY

Radiographic imaging in the critical care unit is an integral part of patient management. Because anteroposterior radiography is one of the first radiographic methods used for patients who have emergent situations that require internal views of the chest and abdomen, the critical care nurse needs to have an understanding of areas to be reviewed, both for patient management and more effective health care team collaboration. Although imaging of patients in the critical care setting can be difficult, the nurse's knowledge regarding the procedure including positioning and imaging needs can be assistive in obtaining a clear, useful image. Medical devices used to maintain physiologic functioning may cause limitations that need to be overcome in performing radiographic procedures. Transport of patients with these devices may also be necessary for tests that require equipment that cannot be transported to the critical care unit. This can be especially difficult for patients with labile vital functioning. The nurse must be attentive to multiple parameters during transport. Radiographic studies are an integral part of critical care patient management. It is imperative that the critical care nurse be cognizant of radiographic studies, and thus be able to collaborate with all health care providers in the administration of quality patient care.

REFERENCES

1. Graat ME, Choi G, Wolthuis EK, et al. The clinical value of daily chest radiographs in a mixed medical-surgical intensive care unit is low. Crit Care 2006. Available at: http://ccforum.com/content/10/1/R11. Accessed May 29, 2009.
2. Silverstein DS, Livingston DH, Elcavage J, et al. The utility of routine chest radiography in the surgical intensive care unit. J Trauma 1993;35:643–6.
3. Price MB, Grant MJ, Welkie K. Financial impact of elimination of routine chest radiographs in a pediatric intensive care unit. Crit Care Med 1999;27:1588–93.
4. Hendrikse KA, Gratama JWC, Hove W, et al. Low value of routine chest radiographs in a mixed medical-surgical ICU. Chest 2007;132(3):823–8. Available at: http://www.chestjournal.org/content/132/3/823.full. Accessed May 18, 2009.
5. Bhagwanjee S, Muckart DJ. Routine daily chest radiography is not indicated for ventilated patients in a surgical ICU. Intensive Care Med 1996;22:1335–8.
6. ACR practice guideline for the performance of pediatric and adult chest radiography. In: Practice guidelines and technical standards. Reston (VA): American College of Radiology; 2006. p. 361–6.
7. Martin GS, Ely EW, Carroll FE, et al. Findings on the portable chest radiograph correlate with fluid balance in critically ill patients. Chest 2002;122(6):2087–95.
8. Khan AN, Al-Jahdali H, Al-Ghanem S, et al. Reading chest radiographs in the critically ill (part I): normal chest radiographic appearance, instrumentation and complications from instrumentation. Ann Thorac Med 2009;4:75–87. Available at: http://www.thoracicmedicine.org/article.asp?issn=1817-1737;year=2009;volume=4; issue=2;spage=75;epage=87;aulast=Khan. Accessed May 18, 2009.
9. Jenkins PF. Making sense of the chest x-ray—a hands-on guide. London: Hodder Arnold; 2005.

10. Filler AG. The history, development, and impact of computed imaging in neurological diagnosis and neurosurgery: CT, MRI, DTI. Nature Precedings 2009. DOI:10.1038/npre.2009.3267.2.

11. Sanders TG, Parsons TW. Radiographic imaging of musculoskeletal neoplasia. Cancer Control 2001;8(3). Available at: http://www.medscape.com/viewarticle/409049_6. Accessed May 18, 2009.

12. Troughton S. Worlds first volume computed tomography (VCT) system, developed by GE Healthcare, scanning patients at Froedtert. Available at: http://www.gehealthcare.com/company/pressroom/releases/pr_release_9722.html. Accessed May 18, 2009.

13. Koichi N, Hironobu K, Takaaki M, et al. Three dimensional imaging by helical volume computed tomography in the evaluation of pathological conditions of bones and joints. Annual Bulletin of Kosei-Nenkin Hospitals 1998;24:15–23.

14. Mattson J, Simon M. The pioneers of NMR and magnetic resonance in medicine: the story of MRI. Jericho (Palestine). New York: Bar-Ilan University Press; 1996.

15. Hodder HF. Bloodless revolution: 21st century surgery. Harv Mag 2000;103(2). Available at: http://harvardmagazine.com/2000/11/bloodless-revolution.html. Accessed May 18, 2009.

16. Russell L. Intraoperative magnetic resonance imaging safety considerations. AORN J 2003;77(3):590–2.

17. Prabhakar R, Haresh KP, Ganesh T, et al. Comparison of computed tomography and magnetic resonance based target volume in brain tumors [serial online]. J Cancer Res Ther 2007;3:121–3. Available at: http://www.cancerjournal.net/text.asp?2007/3/2/121/34694. Accessed May 30, 2009.

18. Yokoi K, Kamiya N, Matsuguma H, et al. Detection of brain metastasis in potentially operable non-small cell lung cancer. Chest 1999;11(3):714–9.

19. Hierholzer J, Luo L, Bittner RC, et al. MRI and CT in the differential diagnosis of pleural disease. Chest 2000;118(3):604–9.

Angiography: From a Patient's Perspective

Leigh Ann McInnis, PhD, RN, FNP-BC[a],*,
Lynn Parsons, DSN, RN, NE-BC[a], Stephen D. Krau, PhD, RN, CNE, CT[b]

KEYWORDS

- Angiography in critical care
- Management of patients presenting with neurologic symptoms
- Evaluation of the cerebral vessels
- Angiographic evaluation of the cerebral and carotid arteries

Patients seen in critical care environments present with many diagnoses and emergent conditions. Patients who present with neurologic symptoms suggestive of stroke, subarachnoid hemorrhage, aneurysm, or transient ischemic attacks require evaluation of the cerebral vessels. During their course of treatment, the majority of these patients require angiographic evaluation of the cerebral and carotid arteries. However, the management of the patient presenting with neurologic symptoms includes procedures that are noninvasive, minimally invasive, and invasive. Each technique has advantages and disadvantages associated with their use. To support and care for patients, critical care nurses should understand the options available.

ANGIOGRAPHY

Angiography is the radiographic visualization of blood vessels after injection of a radiopaque substance, or contrast medium. Thus, simply put, an angiogram is an angiographic image of blood vessels. In many angiographic studies, iodine is used as the contrast medium. Angiography is used to evaluate vessels for blockage or narrowing. The most common types include carotid angiography, cerebral angiography, coronary angiography, aortic angiography, and renal angiography.[1]

DIAGNOSTIC MODALITIES

Many angiographic techniques are used to evaluate the cerebral and carotid vessels. These include conventional cerebral angiography, digital subtraction angiography,

[a] Middle Tennessee State University, School of Nursing, 1500 Greenland Drive, Box # 81, Murfreesboro, TN 37132, USA
[b] Vanderbilt University Medical Center, 314 Godchaux Hall, 461 21st Avenue South, Nashville, TN 37240, USA
* Corresponding author.
E-mail address: lmcinnis@mtsu.edu (L.A. McInnis).

Crit Care Nurs Clin N Am 22 (2010) 51–60
doi:10.1016/j.ccell.2009.10.007

computed tomographic (CT) angiography, and magnetic resonance angiography. In addition to these angiographic approaches, there are other imaging modalities that are less invasive and include CT and magnetic resonance imaging.[1] Although all of these techniques play individual and related roles in the diagnosis and treatment of patients with cerebral and carotid disease, only the role of the angiographic diagnostic modalities will be described in more detail here.

A PATIENT'S PERSPECTIVE

To provide a glimpse into how a patient with neurologic symptoms experiences emergent treatment, coauthor Dr Lynn Parsons recalls her impressions from over 2 decades ago:

> *Imagine being told you had two cranial aneurysms! I was that person. Twenty-four years have passed and my memories of receiving the initial diagnosis and all aspects of treatment remain vivid.*
>
> *I had collapsed after exerting myself doing outdoor activities. My sister recalls that, as I fell to the floor in her living room, I said, "I am stroking out." I have no recall. What I do remember is being globally aphasic initially with right hemiparesis. I could feel my right lower extremity but could not move it. My upper extremity had no sensation or movement. An ambulance arrived minutes later and the paramedic asked, "How old are you?" I answered that I was 21. He said, "No, try again." I said "22." He said, "No, try again." My final response was "23." He said nothing. I was age 29.*
>
> *The fog was clearing and I thought I was acting like a cerebral vascular accident patient. As a registered nurse with a background in neurology, I had seen many stroke patients in practice and cerebral vascular accident was the number-one diagnosis seen on the neuro-rehabilitation floor where I worked. I still could not move my right extremities and I was now experiencing expressive aphasia. I was transported to the local emergency department.*
>
> *The questions continued in the emergency department. Who is the president? What year is it? What time does the clock show? I thought I was doing okay despite visual disturbances. My sister blurted, "Think. You are getting the answers wrong!" In this very tenuous situation, my sense of humor remained intact even though the rest of me seemed to be falling apart. My sister was a schoolteacher serving as principal. Giving incorrect answers caused her great anxiety. I remember thinking I had gotten them right and was somewhat amused with her attitude. I was transported to a regional facility that employed a neurosurgeon. A CT of the head and carotid angiography were completed. Later the diagnosis came: a spontaneous left dissecting carotid aneurysm and a pseudoaneurysm, both at the right internal carotid artery at C-1 level. I was placed on aspirin 5 grain, Pro-Banthine 30 mg, and a heparin drip. I was transferred to a major medical center with medical school affiliations and a team of neurosurgeons.*
>
> *Carotid angiogram was done again confirming the diagnosis. I did not respond to anticoagulant treatment and was experiencing diplopia. The cerebral vascular accident extended to right-sided hemiparesis. My neurosurgeon said I had three options: (1) be treated medically with anticoagulant therapy and possibly have a catastrophic cerebral vascular accident, (2) die, or (3) have a superficial temporal artery to middle cerebral artery anastomosis (STA-MCA bypass).*
>
> *The neurosurgeon went on to say that the STA-MCA bypass could involve drilling two burrs into my skull and doing microsurgery. The less-invasive procedure would decrease the likelihood of postoperative infection and my recovery time.*
>
> *I opted for surgery and made a full recovery. Six weeks after surgery, I returned to work on a surgical-orthopedic unit. The only trace evidence of the entire experience is a subtle seventh cranial nerve (facial) deficit.*

OVERVIEW

This case illustrates now, when a patient presents with emergent neurologic symptoms, many critical decisions must be made as the situation evolves. When the paramedics arrived, they appropriately asked questions to determine if there were focal neurologic deficits or other symptoms, such as nuchal rigidity or headache. Clinical history is an extremely important component of the diagnostic work-up. Next, upon arrival at a local emergency department and after initial stabilization, the patient was transferred to a regional facility with the services of a neurosurgeon. In keeping with the standard of care, the first diagnostic imaging study ordered was a noncontrast CT of the head.[2] The CT scan is considered the foundation for diagnosis in emergent neurologic situations. CT scans can be performed quickly and are extremely sensitive. The main advantages of the CT scan are widespread access and quick acquisition. This imaging technique is usually chosen to exclude or confirm hemorrhage.[3] The CT scan can identify, localize, and quantify an aneurysm or hemorrhage. During the first 24 hours, non–contrast enhanced CT is 90% to 95% sensitive in the identification of subarachnoid hemorrhage.[1,4] After the CT scan was performed, a conventional angiogram was ordered. Even 24 years later, these two imaging approaches remain key components in the assessment of patients with emergent neurologic symptoms.

TYPES OF ANGIOGRAPHY

In addition to conventional cerebral angiography, several other angiographic imaging approaches have been developed or refined in recent years. The approaches described and discussed here include digital subtraction angiography (DSA), CT angiography, and magnetic resonance angiography (MRA).

Conventional Cerebral Angiography

Conventional cerebral angiography, also known as a four-vessel cerebral angiogram, is an invasive test that requires considerable technical skill.[2] During angiography, a catheter is inserted into an artery and advanced until it is in the area of interest for the study. Catheters are usually inserted in the femoral artery to access the arterial system. Once the catheter is in place, an ionic or nonionic iodine compound is injected to enable visualization of blood vessels. Conventional cerebral angiography can be used to detect, diagnose, and treat myocardial ischemia, myocardial infarction, subarachnoid hemorrhages, aneurysms, carotid stenosis, and cerebral ischemia or stroke (**Fig. 1**).

Although conventional cerebral angiography has been considered the diagnostic test of choice for many years, it is rarely performed in the acute setting for diagnostic purposes. This is primarily because of the increasing availability of less-invasive techniques for visualization of intracranial and extracranial vessels.[5] However, if other noninvasive imaging techniques are negative or conflicting, then conventional angiography is performed to evaluate the cerebral circulation for the source of neurologic symptoms.[2]

In patients with suspected intracranial large vessel disease or occlusion, conventional cerebral angiography remains the gold standard. Conventional angiography is more sensitive than noninvasive methods in this group of patients. It also presents the opportunity for treatment that can occur when testing occurs.[3,6] Conventional angiography enables precise calculation of the extent of stenosis, differentiation of arterial occlusion from severe stenosis, assessment of collateral flow patterns, and evaluation of other intracranial and extracranial vessels.[7]

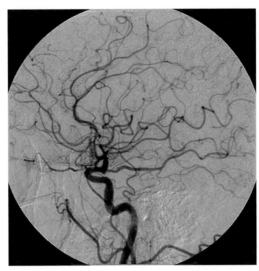

Fig. 1. Cerebral angiogram using iodine-based contrast medium. (*From* Wikipedia: The free encyclopedia. Wikimedia Foundation. Available at: http://en.wikipedia.org/wiki/File: Cerebral_Angiogram_Lateral.jpg. This image is licensed under the GNU Free Documentation License.)

The major drawback of conventional cerebral angiography is the risk of neurologic impairment, such as stroke (0.14%–1.2%) and transient ischemia (0.4%–3%), with a risk of permanent deficits of less than 1%.[3,8] Risks and complications appear to be greater in patients over 55 years of age with atherosclerotic cerebrovascular or cardiovascular disease. Clinically silent embolism has been reported in up to 25% of cerebral angiographic procedures.[3] Because of the skill required to proficiently perform this test, it is best done at a major medical center where such procedures are performed often, thus reducing the risk of complications.[2] In fact, one investigator states that the risk related to conventional cerebral angiogram is inversely proportional to the experience of the individual performing it.[8] In addition to concerns related to neurologic impairment, risks include allergic reaction to contrast, nephrotoxicity, hemorrhage, infections, vascular injuries, dissections, occlusions, and arteriovenous fistulae.[8]

Digital Subtraction Angiography

DSA is similar to conventional cerebral angiography and has many of the same advantages and disadvantages (**Fig. 2**).[9–11] It is an invasive intra-arterial catheter–based technique used to detect, diagnose, and treat intracranial aneurysms, subarachnoid hemorrhages, carotid stenoses, and other neurologic conditions. In conventional angiography, images encompass blood vessels and any overlying structures in the area of study. Although these images provide data regarding anatomic position, they may provide unnecessary additional information without improving visualization of the cerebral blood vessels. In contrast, DSA uses a computer technique to compare images of the body before and after contrast. This enables the radiologist to remove distracting structures, thus providing a clearer image of the area of interest.[9–11]

Computed Tomography Angiography

CT angiography is performed by injecting a bolus of standard contrast through a large-bore intravenous line in the antecubital fossa. Since dye can be seen in the vessels in

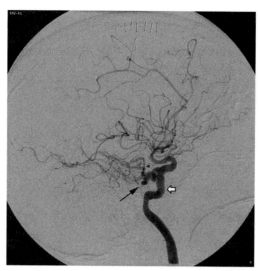

Fig. 2. Digital subtraction angiogram of the internal carotid artery. (*Black arrow*) shows large tortuous vessel. (*white arrow*) indicates the internal carotid artery. (*Courtesy of* Laughlin Dawes, MD.)

the raw images, these data generate three-dimensional views of the circle of Willis and other extracranial cerebral arteries.[3] The contrast dye fills the microvasculature in normal perfused tissue and appears as increased signal intensity on the CT angiographic image. In contrast, dye does not fill the microvasculature in ischemic brain tissue. These areas are easily seen as areas of hypoperfusion and appear dark on CT angiographic images.[3]

CT angiography offers an anatomic representation of the arteries and permits imaging of nearby soft tissue and bony structures. These three-dimensional views enable reasonably accurate measurements of lumen diameter. Images acquired via CT angiography are more sensitive than those acquired via noncontrast CT angiography for the identification of early brain infarct, severe carotid artery disease, and carotid occlusion.[3,12] When compared with intra-arterial cerebral angiography, CT angiography has a sensitivity of 0.77 (95% CI 0.68–0.84) and specificity of 0.95 (95% CI 0.91–0.97) for the diagnosis of 70% to 99% of carotid stenoses.[12] Similarly, when compared with DSA, CT angiography detects severe carotid artery disease, in particular carotid occlusion with a sensitivity and specificity of 97 and 99 percent, respectively.[12]

CT angiography generates beneficial information about complex aneurysms and can augment conventional angiography by showing the connection of the aneurysm to other vessels and the base of the cranium. CT angiography also reveals areas of thrombosis in the aneurysm. CT angiography is a useful imaging technique in the detection of aneurysms greater than 3 mm (95% sensitivity).[8] In some areas, CT angiography has become the first-line imaging choice for the evaluation of subarachnoid hemorrhages. CT angiography is reasonably quick, minimally invasive, and requires fewer resources than does cerebral angiography.[8]

Limitations of CT angiography include decreased sensitivity for detection of aneurysms smaller than 3 mm, relatively poor visualization of perforators, and decreased sensitivity for identification of arteriovenous malformations, dural arteriovenous fistulas, and vasculitis. Similar to conventional angiography, CT angiography depends on the expertise and experience of the individual performing the procedure (**Fig. 3**).[8]

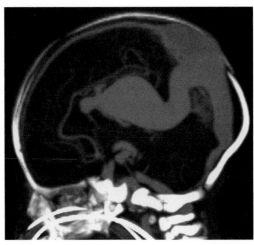

Fig. 3. Projection from a CT angiogram showing an aneurysmal deep venous structure. (*Courtesy of* Laughlin Dawes, MD.)

Magnetic Resonance Angiography

A significant advantage of MRA is that it can be used for imaging in patients with contraindications to the use of contrast. MRA can be performed without contrast using a noninvasive, time-of-flight (TOF-MRA) technique that generates a three-dimensional image produced by the movement of magnetized blood through the area being evaluated (**Fig. 4**).[3,8,11] The disadvantage of this technique is its vulnerability to decay through turbulence and slow blood flow, both of which disrupt the even flow of blood through the vessel lumen. Another MRA technique uses gadolinium contrast for enhanced angiography (CE-MRA). This technique is minimally invasive, but is less dependent on blood flow for quality images of the vasculature and arterial lumen. Although CE-MRA slightly overestimates stenosis in comparison to results of DSA, this disadvantage is outweighed when compared with the risk of stroke associated with DSA.[3,8,11] MRA is recommended for the evaluation and screening of cerebral aneurysms, cerebral venous thrombosis, and arterial dissection.[11,12] It is approximately 95% sensitive for detecting aneurysms measuring at least 3 mm.[8]

However, there are limitations to the use of MR imaging. Patient motion, regardless of imaging technique, can diminish the quality of the image generated. In TOF-MRA, images are dependent on the smooth flow of blood in the vessel being evaluated. Since many patients have stenotic areas in these vessels, signal loss occurs. Although signal loss can indicate stenosis, it can also indicate complete occlusion, making TOF-MRA a poor choice for distinguishing between the two conditions. In comparison, CE-MRA is less sensitive to flow artifacts because of the use of contrast. In fact, CE-MRA can overestimate the degree of carotid stenosis.[11]

COMPARISON

Although CT angiography exposes patients to radiation and iodinated contrast, it has better overall resolution and smaller pixels than MRA, which provides more accurate and detailed images. In addition, CT angiography is less susceptible to artifacts, is quicker, is less likely to show degradation, and generates useful information regarding surrounding anatomy. The issue of sensitivity and specificity of CT angiography as

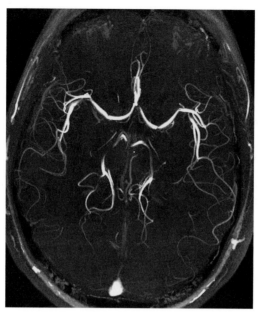

Fig. 4. TOF-MRA showing circle of Willis. (*Courtesy of* S. Barnes.)

compared with MRA is more controversial. While some state that CT angiography is more widely available and has higher sensitivity and specificity,[11] others support MRA as more sensitive and specific.[5,10,13] However, most agree that CT angiography is more portable and less expensive.[5,11] Although a significant amount of research has been conducted on newer, less-invasive imaging approaches, conventional cerebral angiography remains the gold standard that other evaluation techniques are measured against.

EXPERIENCING ANGIOGRAPHY

It is essential to explain the angiography procedure to the patient and his or her family. If the person has a health background, do not assume they will know everything about the procedure. A carotid angiogram is a diagnostic test to determine if there are blockages or narrowing in the carotid arteries that supply blood to the brain.[14]

Preparation for the Procedure

Give the patient written instructions and reinforce these instructions with a verbal explanation. Use illustrations to teach the patient about injection sites and invite questions. Some patients are visual learners and graphics will help them understand information and ask informed questions. Other patients are auditory learners and will learn from the nurse's verbal instructions. Informing the patient of what to expect well ahead of the procedure is prudent.[14,15] Before the procedure, the nurse should:

- Obtain a full health history from the patient.
- Be aware of the patient's current medication regimen.
- Determine if the patient is on warfarin and give a stop date.
- Find out about the patient's known allergies, especially to intravenous pyelogram dye or contrast materials that will be used in the angiography.

- Check on the required preprocedure laboratory work.
- Ensure that the patient is given nothing by mouth a minimum of 6 hours before the procedure.
- Inform the patient that there will be frequent monitoring of vital signs and neurologic and neurovascular checks and that this is normal.
- Explain to the patient that the injection site is usually the femoral artery and that the leg will remain straight during the procedure.
- Advise the patient that it is normal to feel a warm sensation when the dye is injected.

The Actual Procedure

During the procedure, the patient is fully conscious and able to converse with the physician. Sedation is not used to facilitate monitoring of the patient's mental status during the actual procedure.[15] During the process, the care provider should cue the patient on what will occur and be available to answer questions. Ongoing assessment is done, as one caregiver will be with the patient during the entire procedure.[15] In the experience of coauthor Dr Lynn Parsons, the radiologist always stays during angiography procedures and applies pressure post-procedure at the insertion site. The patient can expect:

- Skin preparations with antiseptics, drapes, and a sterile procedure
- Topical anesthesia to numb the entry site (usually groin, but may be neck or elbow area)
- Burning sensation at the injection site from the topical anesthesia
- Placement of the catheter into the artery and then threaded to the carotid arteries while placement is monitored via x-ray
- Pressure at the arterial injection site
- Injection into the arterial site of intravenous pyelogram dye or contrast material, which will flow to the carotid arteries and be monitored with digital pictures taken from many different angles to determine if and where arteries are especially narrow or blocked.
- The angiography to take up to 1 hour
- To have pressure applied to the arterial site for up to 1 hour following the procedure after the catheter is removed

Nurses should inform patients that they will be monitored in the health facility for a minimum of 2 hours and should maintain bed rest for a minimum of 2 to 6 hours with the affected extremity kept straight. Inform the patient that there may be injection site pain and bruising, and that a hematoma may occur. Give the patient and the accompanying family member a phone number to contact if there are unusual symptoms, which include significant pain and/or bleeding at the injection site, paresthesia in the extremities, signs of infection at the injection site, dysarthia, or respiratory difficulties.

PERSONAL EXPERIENCE

Coauthor Dr Parsons recalls her bypass procedure and its aftermath:

Follow-up for the STA-MCA bypass was done at 3 months, 6 months, 1 year, and 2 years after surgery to determine patent bypass. The angiography experience was different each time because of the timing. I was more emotional before surgery because of being unsure of a diagnosis and fearful of what the diagnosis and eventual prognosis would be. Immediately following surgery the standard postoperative angiography to determine cerebral blood flow and patency was done. When the dye was inserted, I felt intense burning, almost what I thought being electrocuted would feel like. I attributed this to the dye transversing a freshly cut vascular system. Follow-up angiography was more predictable and I could brace myself for what was to come. Sharing information (described above) on what to expect is helpful. The nurse caregiver should expect that angiography procedures to be different for each individual.

SUMMARY

Regardless of the procedure used for the detection, evaluation, diagnosis, and management of neurologic emergencies, patient education must be provided. Thus, as nurses in the critical care environment, we must know the steps involved in each of the approaches used to properly prepare our patients. It is important to know the steps involved in each. As part of that preparation, we should explain what patients should expect before, during, and after the procedure has been performed. Examination of the procedure from the patient perspective will help us provide appropriate and empathetic care.

REFERENCES

1. Jandial R, Aryan HE, Hughes SA. U H S, management of intracerebral vascular catastrophes. In: Wilson WC, Grande CM, Hoyt DB, editors, Trauma: critical care, vol. 2. New York: Informa Healthcare USA, Inc; 2007. p. 239–440.
2. Herrmann LL, Zabramski JM. Nonaneurysmal subarachnoid hemorrhage: a review of clinical course and outcome in two hemorrhage patterns. J Neurosci Nurs 2007;39(6):135–42.
3. Oliveira-Filho J, Koroshetz WJ. Neuroimaging of acute ischemic stroke. In: Rose BD, editor. UpToDate. Waltham (MA): UpToDate; 2008.
4. Sunshine JL, Tarr RW. Neuroimaging in neuroemergencies. In: Suarez JI, editor. Critical care neurology and neurosurgery. New York: Humana Press Springer Inc; 2004. p. 123–36.
5. Meschia JF, Brott TG, Hobson RW. Diagnosis and invasive management of carotid atherosclerotic stenosis. Mayo Clin Proc 2007;82(7):851–8.
6. Berg M, Zhang Z, Ikonen A, et al. Multi-detector row CT angiography in the assessment of carotid artery disease in symptomatic patients: comparison with rotational angiography and digital subtraction angiography. AJNR Am J Neuroradiol 2005;26:1022–34.
7. Ehtisham A, Chimowitz MI. Intracranial large artery atherosclerosis. In: Rose BD, editor. UpToDate. Waltham (MA): UpToDate; 2009.
8. Bagley LJ. Aneurysms: all you need to know. Appl Radiol 2009;38(1):6–18.
9. Wagner M, Stenger K. Unruptured intracranial aneurysms: using evidence and outcomes to guide patient teaching. Crit Care Nurs Q 2005;28(4):341–54.
10. Masdeu JC, Irimia P, Asenbaum S, et al. EFNS guideline on neuroimaging in acute stroke: report of an EFNS task force. Eur J Neurol 2006;13:1271–83.
11. Jaff MR, Goldmaker GV, Lev MH, et al. Imaging of the carotid arteries: the role of duplex ultrasonography, magnetic resonance arteriography, and computerized tomographic arteriography. Vasc Med 2008;13:281–92.
12. Wiltrdink JL, Furie KL, Kistler JP. Evaluation of carotid artery stenosis. In: Rose BD, editor. UpToDate. Waltham (MA): UpToDate; 2009.
13. Wardlaw JM, Chappell FM, Best JJ, et al. Non-invasive imaging compared with intra-arterial angiography in the diagnosis of symptomatic carotid stenosis: a meta-analysis. Lancet 2006;367:1503–12.

14. University of Rochester Medical Center Strong Heart and Vascular Center. Available at: http://www.stronghealth.com/services/cardiology/cathep/cathlab/carotidangiogram.cfm. Accessed June 12, 2009.

15. Ignatavicius DD, Workman ML. Medical-surgical nursing patient-centered collaborative care. St. Louis (MO): Saunders Elsevier; 2010.

Nuclear Scan Studies in Critical Care

Leigh Ann McInnis, PhD, RN, FNP-BC[a],*,
Maria A. Revell, DSN, RN, COI[a], Tasha L. Smith, BS[b]

KEYWORDS

- Nuclear • Imaging • Scans • Radioactive
- Radiopharmaceutical • Critical care

Technological improvements during the past decade have led to rapid growth in the field of nuclear medicine. This growth has influenced all health care arenas, including critical care. Patients in critical care have multiple symptoms and diagnoses that may require any number of nuclear scans. For the nurse in critical care, the emergence of new technologies and increasing patient acuity lead to expanded roles and responsibilities.[1]

Nuclear medicine is a division of health care that uses machinery and radioactive isotopes, or radiopharmaceuticals, to assist in the diagnosis and treatment of disease. Nuclear medicine provides information about the function and structure of organs in the body.[1,2] Thus, nuclear scan studies are used in many patient care situations. Patients may have symptoms of, or be diagnosed with conditions such as stroke, Alzheimer's disease, seizures, cancer, coronary artery disease, myocardial infarction, pulmonary emboli, sepsis, hyperthyroidism, heart failure, and many more. The range of nuclear scans available for use is just as broad.[2]

In critical care, nuclear scan studies are used for evaluation and management of many types of patients. Critical care units see a significant number of patients with cardiac diagnoses and related comorbidities. In patients with coronary artery disease (CAD), testing includes coronary angiography or a diverse array of noninvasive tests.[3] Recent research in the field of nuclear medicine has supported the use of noninvasive nuclear myocardial perfusion scans as the best initial imaging studies for the identification of myocardial ischemia.[4] Nuclear myocardial scans include perfusion and gated wall motion imaging. These types of scans encompass many techniques, including single-photon emission computed tomography (SPECT), ECG-gated (GSPECT), technetium 99m (^{99m}Tc)-labeled erythrocyte scintigraphy (also known as a blood pool study), positron emission tomography (PET), and ^{18}F-fluorodeoxyglucose (FDG) PET.[5]

[a] Middle Tennessee State University, 1500 Greenland Drive, PO Box # 81, Murfreesboro, TN 37132, USA
[b] Medtronic, 8200 Coral Sea North East, MVC23, Mounds View, MN 55112, USA
* Corresponding author.
E-mail address: lmcinnis@mtsu.edu (L.A. McInnis).

Crit Care Nurs Clin N Am 22 (2010) 61–74
doi:10.1016/j.ccell.2009.10.008
0899-5885/10/$ – see front matter © 2010 Elsevier Inc. All rights reserved.

The nurse's role in nuclear medicine includes patient education and preparing the patient for the procedure. This can include starting intravenous lines, drawing blood, placing indwelling catheters, providing moderate sedation, and offering physiologic and emotional comfort to the patient during the procedure. Understanding the similarities and differences between various nuclear scan studies is imperative to safe patient care and adequate patient education. Knowledge and awareness of these scans and studies strengthens the critical care nurse's ability to care and advocate for patients.[3] Nurses play a positive and preventive role in nuclear medicine.[6]

NUCLEAR SCAN STUDIES

Nuclear scan studies or radionuclide imaging procedures are noninvasive and usually painless techniques that use radiopharmaceuticals or radiotracers.[5] Radiopharmaceuticals contain either a radionuclide alone, or a radionuclide that is attached to a stable carrier molecule such as a drug, protein, or peptide that concentrates in a particular anatomic area. Radionuclides, or radioisotopes, are unstable isotopes that are radioactive, but become more stable by releasing energy as radiation. The energy released by the radionuclides (called nuclear decay) produces images. This radiation can include gamma-ray photons or positrons, used in PET.[2,7]

In nuclear medicine, each radionuclide has special properties that make it useful for evaluation and management of particular structures or functions. These radionuclides are administered to the patient via oral, inhalation, or intravenous routes, collecting in the organ or tissue to be studied.[1] In a standard planar scan, a gamma camera takes images as gamma rays are released. This creates light photons that are converted into electrical signals. A computer then summarizes and analyzes the signals and integrates them into 2-dimensional images.[8]

Nuclear scans vary from traditional x-rays, ultrasounds, and other diagnostic tests. Ultrasounds, magnetic resonance imaging (MRI), computed tomography (CT), and x-rays are often used to study structure or anatomy. In contrast to these anatomic imaging techniques, nuclear scans are functional imaging techniques that are used to assess hemodynamic processes. This is accomplished by introducing small amounts of radiopharmaceuticals into the body to study organ and tissue function, facilitating early evaluation and management of disease processes (**Table 1**). The organ system being evaluated or explored dictates the radiopharmaceutical used and the route of administration.[5]

Table 1 Commonly used radiopharmaceuticals and their applications			
Radiopharmaceutical/ Radionuclide	Half-Life	Imaging Technique	Target Organ/Tissue
Thallium 201	73 h	SPECT	Myocardium
Tc-99m sestamibi	6.0 h	SPECT	Myocardium, parathyroid, breast, thyroid
Tc-99m tetrofosmin	6.0 h	SPECT	Myocardium, parathyroid
Flourine-18	2.0 h	PET	Glucose metabolism

Abbreviations: PET, positron emission tomography; SPECT, single-photon emission computed tomography; Tc-99m, technetium 99m.

Data from Lecomte R. Biomedical imaging: SPECT and PET. In: Granja C, Leroy C, Stekl I, editors. Proceedings of the Fourth International Summer School on Nuclear Physics Methods and Accelerators in Biology and Medicine 2007;958:115–22.

In the critical care setting, noninvasive nuclear scan studies are useful tools for assessing myocardial perfusion, metabolic function, acute ischemic syndromes, ventricular function, ejection fractions, ventricular volumes, valve function, and risk stratification for myocardial infarct.[9–11] The primary purpose of these studies is to provide an accurate and comprehensive estimate of myocardial perfusion to locate coronary artery stenosis, stratify patient risk, and to enhance patient management decisions.[12–14]

Single-Photon Emission Computed Tomography

Single-photon emission computed tomography (SPECT) is a common nuclear imaging technique. SPECT evaluates heart structure and function.[14] Similar to planar imaging techniques, SPECT nuclear imaging involves the use of gamma-wave-emitting radio-active isotopes. These isotopes are usually bound to a carrier molecule that determines the distribution of the isotope in the body. However, in contrast to the 2-dimensional images produced by planar imaging, SPECT is able to provide 3-dimensional information. To obtain SPECT images, the gamma camera is rotated around the patient and multiple images from multiple angles are obtained.[15] The gamma camera records the photons at multiple projection angles around the patient. At each angle, one static image is acquired.[10] A computer software program then reconstructs the images (**Fig. 1**). SPECT is preferred to planar imaging in scenarios involving organs with complex structure, such as the heart and brain. It is commonly used to detect tumors, metastatic lesions, cerebral perfusion studies, cerebral vascular disease, brain tumors, coronary artery disease, and myocardial muscle damage after infarction.[15]

SPECT is routinely used for myocardial perfusion imaging because it can accurately distinguish patient risk with a high degree of accuracy. It can locate blockages, identifying the location, extent, and severity of perfusion abnormalities.[11] Specifically, SPECT can determine if myocardial infarct has occurred, assess the size of left

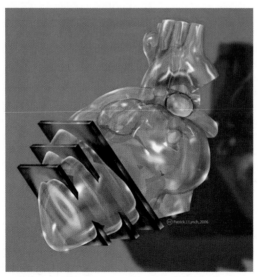

Fig. 1. SPECT nuclear imaging of the heart, short axis views. (*Courtesy of* Patrick J. Lynch, 2006.)

ventricular perfusion defects, the degree or extent of ischemia that can be produced, and the degree of left ventricular dysfunction.[11,16]

SPECT can determine perfusion defect size (PDS) after a myocardial infarct. This information can be used to predict patient outcome. Research shows that if the resting left ventricular perfusion defect is 20% or greater, there is a considerably higher mortality rate than with smaller-sized defects. SPECT can accurately classify patient risk in stable patients post myocardial infarct by assessing PDS, the degree of inducible ischemia, and the extent of left ventricular dysfunction. This allows patients to be discharged from the hospital earlier, minimizing the use of expensive hospital resources and limiting risks to patients inherent to the hospital environment. Outpatient testing and evaluation can be accomplished subsequently as clinically indicated.[16] The radiopharmaceuticals commonly used for SPECT are labeled with gamma-emitting radionuclides and include ^{99m}Tc tetrofosmin, ^{99m}Tc sestamibi, or thallium-201 (^{201}Tl). Each of these radionuclides has unique properties that make them appropriate for specific purposes.

Thallium-201

The original agent used in myocardial perfusion studies was [201]Tl. It is considered the "gold standard" for viability assessment among single-photon agents. This radionuclide was initially used as a perfusion tracer because of its high (approximately 80%) first-pass extraction (or uptake) from the blood into the myocardial cell. This uptake is relatively unaffected by ischemia or hypoxia and is proportional to coronary blood flow.[12] [201]Tl uptake by cardiac cells is dependent on an intact cell membrane. Thus, delivery of the tracer to the cardiac cell is an indicator of regional perfusion and cardiac viability. This radionuclide, because of its rapid uptake by cardiac cells, does not require a carrier molecule.[17]

After injection with ^{201}Tl, the radionuclide is rapidly redistributed. Redistribution permits a single injection for both stress and rest images. This means that after its initial uptake by the cardiac cell, there is a steady exchange between the cardiac cell and the extracellular compartment. Further uptake of thallium from the blood into the cell continues. This process of redistribution can begin as early as 20 minutes following its introduction into the body. Clinically, this necessitates the use of stress imaging, obtained 5 to 10 minutes after injection of ^{201}Tl, followed by late redistribution imaging 4 hours or longer after injection.[17–19]

Defects identified during stress imaging (an active state) can represent regional ischemia or nonviable myocardium.[3] Areas of inadequate perfusion appear as "cold spots," thus pinpointing sites of myocardium at risk. Redistribution images reflect the "resting" state of myocardial perfusion. At rest, thallium may be seen filling areas of the myocardium that were underperfused during initial imaging because of ischemia. This represents a reversible defect. In areas of the heart where irreversible damage has occurred, there is no resolution of the defect with rest imaging. This is indicative of a fixed defect. These imaging results provide information regarding areas of inducible ischemia at risk for future infarct, areas already irreversibly damaged, and the size of any defect. A positive test demonstrates reversible ischemia.[3,20]

There are limitations to the use of [201]Tl. Delayed images frequently underestimate myocardial viability, which often make it necessary to obtain a third set of images either 30 minutes after a second tracer injection or 24 hours after the stress injection.[17,18] [201]Tl emits low photon energy and has a longer physical half-life, which restricts dose and results in decreased image quality (**Table 2**).[19]

Table 2
Radionuclides: single-photon emission computed tomography

	Advantages	Disadvantages
[201]Tl	Myocardial uptake is proportional to flow. Redistribution allows a single injection for both stress and rest images. It is considered the "gold standard" for viability assessment among single-photon agents. Superior image quality especially in obese or female patients.[12,14,17–19]	Low photon energy results in more scatter and soft tissue attenuation. Longer physical half-life limits the allowable dose, which reduces image quality. Because of rapid redistribution with this agent, camera scheduling can be challenging. In comparison with other agents, use relatively high doses.[12,19]
[99m]Tc (tetrofosmin or sestamibi)	Ability to measure resting left ventricular function. Myocardial uptake is proportional to flow rather than viability. Stable retention of tracer (minimal redistribution), minimal cardiac washout, which allows timing flexibility. Useful in acute chest pain because patient can be injected with sestamibi immediately and imaged several hours later. Simultaneous perfusion and function assessment possible.[12,19]	In areas of low blood flow, viable myocardial tissue may be identified as scar tissue. Myocardial uptake is slower than with thallium. In comparison with sestamibi, tetrofosmin causes less hepatic interference, which allows patients to undergo imaging sooner after injection. Tc-99m tetrofosmin stress imaging –15 minutes after injection; Tc-99m sestamibi stress imaging –30–60 minutes after injection. Tc-99m sestamibi images obtained after rest injection require a delay of 45 to 90 minutes to permit hepatic clearance, whereas Tc-99m tetrofosmin require delay of only 30 minutes. Agents are comparable in identifying patients with CAD and detecting stenosed coronary vessels. Tc-99m agents have similar diagnostic sensitivity to ^{201}Tl, but improved image quality results in dramatically improved specificity (ie, reduced false positives).[12,19,21]

Abbreviations: Tc-99m, technetium 99m; ^{201}Tl, thallium 201.

Technetium-99m Radiotracers

There are two additional radiotracers commonly used in SPECT imaging, technetium-99m (^{99m}Tc) tetrofosmin and ^{99m}Tc sestamibi. Studies with ^{99m}Tc agents reveal improved gamma camera imaging and resolution compared with [201]Tl. These tracers show limited redistribution and short half-life in comparison with [201]Tl.[17,18]

The uptake of ^{99m}Tc tracers within cardiac cells is dependent upon the presence of intact electrochemical gradients across the cardiac cell membrane. The uptake of ^{99m}Tc sestamibi across the myocardial cell membrane is accomplished via passive diffusion (in contrast to ^{201}Tl). Because these tracers accumulate in myocardial tissue in a degree proportional to myocardial blood flow, uptake of these tracers by the myocardium generally corresponds to myocardial perfusion. If these agents are injected during or shortly after resolution of chest pain, areas of ischemic myocardium demonstrate reduced radioactive counts.[14]

In contrast to ^{201}Tl, these radiotracers show limited redistribution within the myocardium. This is especially useful in patients with acute chest pain, as accurate information about myocardial perfusion at the time of injection is provided even if imaging is delayed several hours. Rest imaging using ^{99m}Tc can estimate the degree of myocardium at risk during acute coronary artery occlusion, after coronary revascularization and final infarct size.[14,16,22] [99m]Tc tracers also allow the concurrent assessment of perfusion and function. [99m]Tc tetrofosmin and ^{99m}Tc sestamibi are comparable in their ability to identify patients with stenosis and CAD.[19]

Similar to other radiopharmaceuticals and radiotracers, ^{99m}Tc agents have limitations (see **Table 2**). In areas of low blood flow, viable myocardium may be misidentified as scar tissue, emphasizing that uptake is proportional to flow, not viability. However, since no significant redistribution of these agents occurs, separate stress and rest injections are necessary. In comparison, ^{99m}Tc tetrofosmin causes less hepatic interference that ^{99m}Tc sestamibi, allowing patient scans to occur sooner after injection (15 minutes as compared with 30 to 60 minutes).[19]

Dual-isotope Imaging

The dual-isotope imaging approach combines a resting thallium injection and subsequent scan with the injection of either ^{99m}Tc sestamibi or tetrofosmin during stress. This approach generates improved laboratory outcomes and patient satisfaction owing to diminished imaging time. With this technique, a resting injection of ^{201}Tl is given first. This injection is followed by imaging approximately 15 minutes later. Next, the patient is stressed and the radionuclide ^{99m}Tc sestamibi or tetrofosmin is injected. GSPECT imaging is performed 15 to 45 minutes later. Using this technique (exercise-stress), the complete procedure takes only 90 minutes. However, if myocardial viability is an issue, then delayed ^{201}Tl images can be obtained either before or 24 hours after stress. This approach takes advantage of the benefits of both ^{99m}Tc and ^{201}Tl radionuclides.[18]

Gated Single-Photon Emission Computed Tomography

Similar to a standard SPECT scan, a GSPECT procedure requires that a radionuclide, or tracer, be injected. This tracer is then taken up by the cardiac cells in the left ventricle. Similar to SPECT, a gamma camera records the photons at multiple projection angels around the patient. However, instead of one static image, several dynamic images spanning the length of the cardiac cycle are acquired at equal intervals during a GSPECT. Although 8 frames is sufficient for image quality, collecting a greater number of frames improves image resolution. Conversely, an increase in the number of frames collected increases study and processing time. However, as technology has improved, a greater number of frames can be acquired without increases in scan duration or processing time.[10] Any tracer can be used in a GSPECT procedure; however, ^{99m}Tc sestamibi or tetrofosmin provide higher count density, which ensures more consistent high-quality gated images than those obtained with [201]Tl.[18]

A primary advantage to a GSPECT scan is that it results in two datasets. The first is a standard dataset used to evaluate perfusion. The second is a GSPECT dataset used to assess function.[18] The ECG-gated myocardial perfusion GSPECT is a modern technique for the combined evaluation of myocardial perfusion and left ventricular function within a single study. Further, the images provided by a GSPECT provide information related to ventricular ejection fraction, wall motion, wall thickening, and systolic and diastolic volumes. This technique can be used to estimate the remaining function after infarct.[10]

In the critical care patient, surgical interventions for various cardiac and noncardiac conditions are common. GSPECT is an effective tool to assess preoperative risk and may predict perioperative cardiac events. In patients with chronic coronary artery disease and left ventricular dysfunction, restoration of blood flow using surgical revascularization is a principal component of treatment. With surgery, dysfunctional but viable myocardium may be reversible. In contrast, surgery is not indicated for myocardium that has suffered a true infarct. In fact, surgery in this patient group is not only unnecessary, it is associated with significant surgical morbidity and mortality. Thus, before intervention, differentiation between viable and nonviable myocardium is critical. GSPECT can also assess functional changes after coronary revascularization by comparing left ventricular function before and after the procedure an increase in the left ventricular ejection fraction, a decrease in end-systolic volume, and improved contractile function of the myocardium indicate functional improvement.[10] GSPECT is considered one of the more prognostic imaging techniques.[23]

Blood Pool Studies

During a blood pool study, the patient's red blood cells (RBCs) are radiolabeled and ECG-gated cardiac scintigraphy is obtained. This may include single or multiple measurements of left and/or right ventricular function. This procedure is also referred to as gated equilibrium radionuclide ventriculography (RVG), equilibrium-gated radionuclide angiography (ERNA), gated cardiac blood-pool imaging, multigated acquisition (MUGA), or gated equilibrium radionuclide angiography (RNA).[24]

Blood pool studies measure heart function, valve function, ejection fraction, and cardiac chambers. Blood pool studies generate images of the beating heart that can be presented as a single, composite cardiac cycle. This procedure assesses cardiac wall motion, cardiac chamber size, chamber structure, and ventricular systolic and diastolic function. Blood pool studies may be performed at rest, during exercise, or after intervention.[24] The information gathered during this procedure helps predict long-term and short-term survival after infarct.[10]

Positron Emission Tomography

The use of positron emission tomography (PET) scans is evolving. Although PET was primarily developed for research in the brain, it is now more widely used. Some of the applications include the detection of cancer, response to cancer treatment, and evaluation of neurologic and neurodegenerative disorders. In addition, PET imaging has been extensively studied and used in the diagnosis of coronary artery disease.[5]

A PET scan is an imaging technique that uses positively charged particles to detect subtle changes in the body's metabolism and chemical activities.[8] An advantage to this noninvasive approach is the ability to assess perfusion and metabolism (viability) simultaneously.[17] A PET scan provides an image of the function of a particular area of the body rather than its structure. Because functional change precedes structural change, PET scans can potentially detect abnormalities earlier than conventional imaging techniques (**Fig. 2**).[17]

During a PET scan, a positron-producing radioisotope is given to the patient by the intravenous route. The primary radiopharmaceuticals used in cardiac applications of PET include Rb-82 or N-13 ammonia to evaluate myocardial perfusion and F-18 fluorodeoxyglucose (^{18}F-FDG) for myocardial viability.[25] The radiotracer releases positrons that leave the nucleus of an atom and travel short distances through surrounding tissue, losing energy as they collide with other molecules. As the

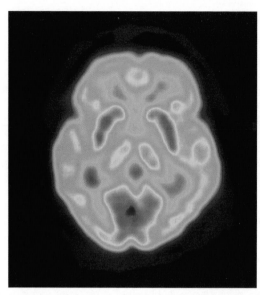

Fig. 2. Typical PET acquisition of the brain. This is an image taken from a typical PET acquisition of the brain. Red areas show more accumulated radioactivity and blue areas are portions where low to no activity was accumulated. This illustrates the appearance of a typical PET image.

positrons begin to stop moving, they combine with electrons. The mass of the positron and electron is converted to energy, or radiation, by the process of annihilation. The energy produced is disseminated as two high-energy gamma rays or photons that travel outward in opposite directions. The PET scanner surrounding the patient detects the gamma rays. A detector in the opposite direction looks for a matching photon. If two matching photons are recorded within a few moments of each other, the detectors note the coincidence. When the scan is complete, overlapping areas signify more highly concentrated areas of radioactivity. The more coincidences that are detected, the more accurate the calculation will be (p381).[8]

PET studies evaluate myocardial function, metabolic changes, and myocardial perfusion. They establish risk and prognosis in cardiac patients by establishing myocardial viability. PET scans assess for coronary artery disease by determining the extent of heart muscle metabolism compared with flow in the myocardium.[8,15]

PET scans allow exploration of functional processes with higher sensitivity and specificity than SPECT. This is primarily because of coincidence detection, but also because some of the radionuclides used in PET scans are organic. Organic radionuclides can be introduced without altering biologic activity. Thus, PET radiotracers can be used to explore virtually any biologic process without interfering with normal function.[15] However, PET scans are not widely available and thus not as accessible as SPECT and GSPECT. PET scans are also limited by their high cost and long-term commitment limitations (**Box 1**).

18F-Fluorodeoxyglucose Positron Emission Tomography

Clearly, PET is a functional imaging technique with significant clinical applications. A cardiac PET scan that uses ^{18}F-fluorodeoxyglucose (^{18}F-FDG) can provide additional information in the selection of patients who present with coronary artery disease and/or diminished left ventricular function. This information helps determine which individuals might benefit from coronary artery revascularization.[25] ^{18}F-FDG PET scan uses FDG as a radiotracer.[8] Although other positron emitters are available to evaluate myocardial viability with PET, other positron emitters have short half-lives that require on-site cyclotron. This is costly and is not widely available in most institutions. In contrast, ^{18}F-FDG is more widely available. This is because of its increased use in oncology and its relatively long half-life when compared with other positron emitters. ^{18}F-FDG is an analog of glucose that allows noninvasive evaluation of glucose metabolism. Because glucose metabolism is an ATP-dependent process, it requires viable myocardial cells. Normal myocardium with normal perfusion has normal glucose uptake. In contrast, areas of infracted myocardium have reduced perfusion and glucose uptake. Hibernating myocardium has reduced perfusion under stress, but normal glucose use. Thus, FDG-PET can distinguish ischemic but still viable myocardium from scar tissue.[19,27]

However, cardiac cells use fatty acids and glucose to meet energy needs. Thus, although FDG uptake in the myocardium indicates viable myocardium, a lack of uptake does not necessarily signify nonviable tissue. To ensure primarily glucose metabolism in the myocardium at the time of tracer injection and scanning, the patient should be fasting for 6 to 12 hours before administration of a standard glucose load (oral or intravenous). This produces rising plasma glucose and insulin levels causing glucose to be the preferred energy source for the cardiac cell. This is an acceptable approach for nondiabetic patients.[25]

PET scans are similar to SPECT scans in their use of radioactive materials. However, in contrast to SPECT, which directly measures gamma radiation, PET scans produce an image drawn from two matching photons. This process is called coincidence imaging. This type of imaging process produces an image with a higher resolution than an image using a SPECT scan.[28] SPECT scans, however, are significantly less expensive than PET scans.[19]

CRITICAL CARE NURSING RESPONSIBILITIES

Critical care nurses need to provide information to patients regarding preparation for tests and test procedures. Many patients and families will be concerned by the use of terms such as "nuclear," "radiopharmaceutical," "radionuclide," and "radioisotope." Therefore, nurses will need to be prepared to answer questions from patients and their families regarding the advantages and disadvantages of various imaging techniques. Remind patients that nuclear medicine procedures are used to acquire information that would otherwise not be available, or would require invasive tests or surgery.[5] Radiopharmaceuticals are safe for use. Similar to any other medication, radiopharmaceuticals are tested carefully by the US Food and Drug Administration before approval for use in patients. The risk of reaction is approximately 2 to 3 incidents per 100,000 injections. Of these reactions, more than 50% are rashes. In comparison, there are approximately 2000 to 3000 reactions per 100,000 injections of x-ray contrast media. In patients undergoing exercise stress tests, the procedure is associated with a complication rate of 1 to 5 cardiac events per 10,000 patients tested. Approximately 4 of 10,000 patients have a myocardial infarction and 1 of 10,000 patients die of cardiac causes during the test.[4]

Patient Education for Gated and Single-Photon Emission Computed Tomography

Indications for radionuclide myocardial perfusion imaging include assessment of presence and degree of coronary artery disease, assist in management of patients with known disease, and assess myocardial viability and hibernation related to possible

---

Box 1
Nuclear scan studies

SPECT

Clinical use and advantages

- Radionuclides used for SPECT have longer half-life
- Procedure more readily available to the medical community
- Evaluates heart structure, function providing data regarding metabolic and diastolic function
- Well-validated ability to assess perfusion and viability
- Identifies blockages in the coronary arteries, predicts risk for myocardial infarct, assesses prognosis, and determines if myocardial infarct has occurred
- Assesses patient condition after revascularization
- Size of perfusion defect predicts outcome
- Results are reproducible
- Assesses left ventricular size qualitatively[16]

Diagnostic considerations

- Use of radionuclides presents potential risks of adverse reactions and radiation exposure (dependent on radionuclide and dose)
- Limited imaging area/limited image detail; soft tissue attenuation artifacts
- Imaging delays—must give the radionuclide time to reach target tissue
- Specificity depends on quality control of laboratory and specialty trained readers
- Specialized equipment and personnel needed[26]

GSPECT

Clinical use and advantages

- Assesses systolic function
- Measures ventricular wall motion, wall thickening, volume, and ejection fraction
- Used to assess effects of reperfusion techniques on infarct size and clinical outcome
- Used to monitor changes in stress-induced perfusion pattern after noninvasive interventions
- Estimates residual function after myocardial infarction
- Provides risk stratification and survival prediction
- Useful in preoperative risk assessment of patients undergoing major noncardiac surgery
- May predict perioperative cardiac events
- One of the more prognostic imaging techniques[10,22,23]

Diagnostic considerations

- Use of radionuclides presents potential risk related to exposure (dependent on radionuclide and dose) and adverse reaction
- Soft tissue attenuation can negatively impact images
- Scanning with 201Tl does not produce high-quality images—best to use 99mTc (tetrofosmin or sestamibi)[10,22,23]

Blood pool studies

Clinical use and advantages

- Measures heart function; valve function, cardiac chambers
- Measures ejection fraction
- Helps predict long-term and short-term survival after myocardial infarct[24]

Diagnostic considerations

- Certain medications and chronic medical conditions can decrease red blood cell labeling (example: chronic kidney disease)
- Incorrect patient positioning can cause the ejection fraction to be inaccurately calculated[24]

PET

Clinical use and advantages

- Important tool for diagnosis of coronary artery disease and establishing prognosis
- Evaluates heart function, metabolic changes, and perfusion
- Evaluates damage to cardiac cells after myocardial infarct and helps guide treatment
- PET images have higher sensitivity than SPECT images[2,25]

Diagnostic considerations

- Not widely available, making it relatively inaccessible, high costs, long time commitment, radiation exposure, specificity dependent on quality control of laboratory and trained readers
- Low specificity in presence of left bundle branch block (LBBB)
- Standardized metabolic conditions have to be present to achieve reproducible results[19,27]

FDG-PET

Clinical use and advantages

- Detects the enhancement of glucose metabolism under ischemic conditions
- FDG has moderately long physical half-life
- Can distinguish ischemic but still viable myocardium from scar tissue
- Sensitivity is greater than SPECT and GSPECT techniques
- FDG-PET may be more useful for identifying appropriate patients for revascularization
- Can predict long-term survival[25]

Diagnostic considerations

- Standardized metabolic conditions have to be present to achieve reproducible results, which can be especially difficult to achieve in diabetic patients
- Myocardial use of glucose is variable, requiring good patient preparation
- Without protocol modification, suboptimal image quality is generated in many diabetic patients[25]

revascularization.[29] Depending on the purpose of the study, there may be variations in patient preparation.

In the general population, nuclear myocardial perfusion studies usually include a stress test (exercise), a resting scan, and a poststress scan. In critical care patients, the stress test may be accomplished using a pharmacologic agent rather than physical exercise. Regardless of methodology, the initial responsibility is to provide the patient with information about the procedure and the risks, benefits, and expected impact on subsequent care. Once the patient validates understanding of the information, it is important to have the patient provide written informed consent for the procedure. Although the risks to patients undergoing pharmacologic stress versus exercise stress are slightly less, patients should still be provided accurate information.[6,29]

Preparation for a SPECT or GSPECT includes abstaining from caffeine for 12 to 24 hours before the study. This time span allows for the various imaging protocols (dynamic exercise or pharmacologic). Recommendations vary by institution and planned procedure, but fasting up to 4 hours before the procedure may be recommended.[4,29] Patients should be instructed that intravenous (IV) access will be necessary.

The next step in the process is to determine the purpose of the test. If the objective is to assess for the presence of coronary artery disease, all patient medications that may interfere with the procedure response should be considered.[4,29] However, if the purpose of the test is to measure response to treatment, then patients should continue their prescribed cardiac medications as directed. Insulin usage should be addressed on a patient-by-patient basis. Before the procedure, cardiovascular history and physical examination should be completed with baseline vital signs and 12-lead ECG.[4]

A procedure manual containing step-by-step instructions for each procedure should be available to the nurse on the critical care unit. This manual should contain quality control procedures for all equipment and radiation safety measures. This manual should be updated and reviewed by all key stakeholders on a regular basis.[4]

Patient Education for Positron Emission Tomography

Although other radiopharmaceuticals are used in cardiac procedures, for the assessment of myocardial viability, ^{18}F-FDG is the most commonly used. This is in part because of its increasing usages and applications in addition to its relatively long half-life.[25] Because ^{18}F-FDG has a chemical structure similar to glucose, it is important to ensure uptake of ^{18}F-FDG by the myocardium. To ensure predominantly glucose metabolism in nondiabetic patients at the time of injection, it is common to fast the patient for 6 to 12 hours and then administer a standardized glucose load. This produces rising plasma glucose and insulin causing glucose to be the preferred energy source of the myocardium.[8,25] Typical protocols used in nondiabetic patient populations result in suboptimal image quality in diabetic patients. In patients who are diabetic or glucose-intolerant, adjustments may be required to diet and medications on (and/or before) PET-scan day. These modifications should be made on a case-by-case basis. Regardless, in most institutions, blood glucose levels are required to be less than 150 mg/dL before injection.[8,25]

Generally, before scan initiation, fasting blood glucose is checked. If it is less than 100 mg/dL, 100-g glucose is administered followed by repeat blood glucose measurement 30 to 45 minutes later. If glucose is less than 140 mg/dL, FDG will be ordered. If blood glucose is higher than 140 mg/dL, then IV boluses of regular insulin are ordered to decrease blood glucose below 140 mg/dL. FDG will be ordered once this level is reached. The protocol for IV glucose loading should be available on your unit.[25] Once the tracer is injected, patients generally wait 30 to 60 minutes for uptake. The scan itself may take from 15 to 120 minutes. There should be no side effects associated with the radiotracer used in the scan.[8]

General Responsibilities

Regardless of procedure, before initiation, the nurse should carefully assess historical data. This should include review of the following: consent, medications, allergies, any potential drug-drug interactions, symptoms, cardiac risk factors, comorbidities, and prior procedures. Vital signs should be obtained with special attention to cardiac rhythm. Marked heart rate variability should be noted, as it may impact testing and interpretation. A 12-lead ECG is often requested before a scan. During imaging, the nurse may be expected to comfort the patient, periodically check vital signs, and monitor blood glucose.[6]

SUMMARY

The field of nuclear cardiology has grown significantly over the past decade. This is a reflection of the value seen by providers in these safe and effective procedures. Nuclear scan studies are noninvasive and versatile in their usefulness. These studies assist in determining the likelihood of future cardiac events, guide approaches to revascularization, and assist in evaluation of the adequacy of revascularization procedures.[29] Critical thinking and decision-making abilities are two key requirements for nurses in the critical care environment. Knowledge and understanding of the nuclear scan studies indicated for patients help nurses advocate for those in their care.

REFERENCES

1. Goodhart J, Page J. Radiology nursing. Orthop Nurs 2007;26:36–9.
2. Committee on State of the Science of Nuclear Medicine, National Research Council. Advancing nuclear medicine through innovation. Washington, DC: The National Acadamies Press; 2007.
3. Krause RS, Koenig BO. Review of cardiac tests. Emedicine 2008. Available at: http://emedicine.medscape.com/article/811577-overview. Accessed May 30, 2009.
4. Heston TF. Myocardial ischemia—nuclear medicine and risk stratification. Emedicine 2008. Available at: http://emedicine.medscape.com/article/352401-media. Accessed May 29, 2009.
5. Society of Nuclear Medicine. What is nuclear medicine? Reston (VA): Society of Nuclear Medicine; 2004.
6. Vijayakumar V, Briscoe EG, Vijayakumar S. Role of nurses in daily nuclear medicine. Internet J Nucl Med 2007;3(2). Available at: http://www.ispub.com/ostia/index.php?xmlFilePath=journals/ijnuc/vol3n2/nurses.xml. Accessed April 28, 2009, from Academic Search Premier database.
7. Jacobson JA. Radionuclide scanning. In: The Merck manuals online medical library for healthcare professionals. Whitehouse Station (NJ): Merck & Co, Inc; 2008. Available at: http://www.merck.com/mmpe/sec22/ch329/ch329f.html?qt=spect&alt=sh; 2008. Accessed May 25, 2009.
8. Lobrano MD, Singha P. Positron emission tomography in oncology. Clin J Oncol Nurs 2003;7:379–85.
9. Bax JJ, Kim CY, Poldermans D, et al. Cardiac applications of FDG imaging with PET and SPECT. In: Delbeke D, Martin WH, Patton JA, editors. Practical FDG imaging. New York: Springer Inc; 2002. p. 75–102.
10. Paul AK, Nabi HA. Gated myocardial perfusion SPECT: basic principles, technical aspects and clinical applications. J Nucl Med Technol 2004;32:179–87.
11. Pirich C, Graf S, Behesthi M. Diagnostic and prognostic impact of nuclear cardiology in the management of acute coronary syndromes and acute myocardial infarction. Imaging Decisions MRI 2004;8:9–16. Available at: http://www.wiley.com/bw/journal.asp?ref=1433-3317.

12. Holly TA, Kansal P. Basic properties of myocardial perfusion. In: Rose BD, editor. UpToDate. Waltham (MA): UpToDate; 2008. Available at: http://www.uptodate.com/home/index.html.

13. Weiner DA. Advantages and limitations of different stress testing modalities. In: Rose BD, editor. UpToDate. Waltham (MA): UpToDate; 2009. Available at: http://www.uptodate.com/home/index.html.

14. Azar RR, Hellar GV. Acute rest radionuclide myocardial perfusion imaging for the evaluation of suspected non-ST elevation acute coronary syndrome. In: Rose BD, editor. UpToDate. Waltham (MA): UpToDate; 2009. Available at: http://www.uptodate.com/home/index.html.

15. Lecomte R. Biomedical imaging: SPECT and PET. In: Granja C, Leroy C, Stekl I, editors. Proceedings of the Fourth International Summer School on nuclear physics methods and accelerators in biology and medicine 2007;958:115–22.

16. Pirich C, Rettenbacher L. Diagnostic and prognostic impact of nuclear medicine in the management of acute chest pain. Imaging Decisions MRI 2006;10:16–21. Available at: http://www.wiley.com/bw/journal.asp?ref=1433-3317.

17. Soman P, Udelson JE. Assessment of myocardial viability by nuclear imaging in coronary heart disease. In: Rose BD, editor. UpToDate. Waltham (MA): UpToDate; 2009. Available at: http://www.uptodate.com/home/index.html.

18. DePasquale E. Role of myocardial perfusion imaging in managing CAD. Medscape Radiology 2003;4(1). Available at: http://www.medscape.com/viewarticle/449487. Accessed May 25, 2009.

19. Occleshaw CJ, Greaves SC, Gerber IL. Cardiac testing. In: Sidebotham D, McKee A, Gillham M, et al, editors. Cardiothoracic critical care. New York: Elsevier Health Sciences; 2007. p. 73–86.

20. Underwood SR, Anagnostopoulos C, Cerqueira M, et al. Myocardial perfusion scintigraphy: the evidence. Eur J Nucl Med Mol Imaging 2004;31:261–91.

21. Shea MJ. Radionuclide imaging. In: The Merck manuals online medical library for healthcare professionals. Whitehouse Station (NJ): Merck & Co, Inc; 2009. Available at: http://www.merck.com/mmpe/sec07/ch070/ch070i.html. Accessed May 25, 2009.

22. Rendl G, Altenberger J, Pirich C. Cardiac imaging in acute coronary syndromes and acute myocardial infarction—an update. Imaging Decisions MRI 2006;10:21–31.

23. Miller DD, Shaw LJ. Coronary artery disease: diagnostic and prognostic models for reducing patient risk. J Cardiovasc Nurs 2006;21:S2–16.

24. Scheiner J, Sinusas A, Wittry MD, et al. Society of Nuclear Medicine procedure guideline for gated equilibrium radionuclide ventriculography. In: Society of Nuclear Medicine procedure guidelines manual. Reston (VA): Society of Nuclear Medicine; 2002. Available at: http://interactive.snm.org/index.cfm?PageID=772.

25. Ghesani M, DePuey EG, Rozanski A. Role of F-18 FDG positron emission tomography (PET) in the assessment of myocardial viability. Echocardiography 2005; 22:165–77.

26. Gebker R, Schwitter J, Fleck E, et al. How we perform myocardial perfusion with cardiovascular magnetic resolution. J Cardiovasc Magn Reson 2007;9:539–47.

27. Janssen CHC, Kuijpers D, Oudkerk M. MR perfusion imaging for the detection of myocardial ischemia. Imaging Decisions MRI 2004;8:13–7. Available at: http://www.wiley.com/bw/journal.asp?ref=1433-3317.

28. Bonte FJ, Harris TS, Hynan LS, et al. Tc99m HMPAO SPECT in the differential diagnosis of the dementias with histopathologic confirmation. Clin Nucl Med 2006;31:376–8.

29. Anagnostopoulos C, Harbinson M, Kelion A, et al. Procedure guidelines for radionuclide myocardial perfusion imaging. Heart 2004;90(Suppl 1):i1–10 d.

Allergy Skin Testing: What Nurses Need to Know

Stephen D. Krau, PhD, RN, CNE, CT [a],*,
Leigh Ann McInnis, PhD, RN, FNP-BC [b], Lynn Parsons, DSN, RN, NE-BC [b]

KEYWORDS

• Skin tests • Patch test • Allergy • Allergy testing

Skin testing is a common procedure in any clinical setting, and a practice that all health care providers have experienced as either the tester or the individual being tested for allergies, or as a screen for infectious diseases such as tuberculosis. Critical care nurses will encounter skin testing in the inpatient and outpatient settings primarily to test for patient allergies to environmental factors, or allergies to certain medications. Testing for allergies should always follow a thorough history and physical examination, as the skin tests are used to confirm or exclude allergies. At present there is a great deal of controversy about standard practices surrounding the different tests, and although there is some current research on skin testing, there is overall a lack of evidenced-based standard protocols for administering and interpreting the results of skin tests. There are many patient variants, and testing variants that can impact the results of the tests as well as the reliability and usefulness of the results. Information about allergy tests and testing will lead the nurse toward important considerations when administering, interpreting, and teaching the patient about allergy skin testing.

The first documented skin test is credited to Charles H. Blackley, a physician with chronic allergic rhinitis.[1] He abraided his skin with a lancet and applied wet lint soaked in grass pollen to the area, which resulted in severe itching and a large cutaneous response.[1,2] Today, there is not much departure from the principles that were first used by Blackley. Awareness of the controversies and the positive and negative aspects of the predictive value of any skin test are paramount. In addition, skin testing must be considered with regard to the patient's history and physical status. The interpretation of the test is contingent on many factors. Factors that warrant consideration include the type of skin testing, the device used to test the skin, the placement of the

[a] Vanderbilt University Medical Center, 314 Godchaux Hall, 461 21st Avenue South, Nashville, TN 37240, USA
[b] Middle Tennessee State University, School of Nursing, 1500 Greenland Drive, Box # 81, Murfreesboro, TN 37132, USA
* Corresponding author.
E-mail address: stephen.krau@vanderbilt.edu (S.D. Krau).

Crit Care Nurs Clin N Am 22 (2010) 75–82
doi:10.1016/j.ccell.2009.10.009
0899-5885/10/$ – see front matter © 2010 Elsevier Inc. All rights reserved.
ccnursing.theclinics.com

test on the patient's body, the substance being used to test the skin, the potential interferences such as medications that may suppress the skin response, and parameters relating to the interpretation of the tests.

METHODS OF SKIN TESTING

Skin tests may be performed using either a prick or puncture (percutaneous), and can be performed by intradermal (intracutaneous) techniques or through patch testing, in which the extract is applied directly to the skin (epicutaneous). Intradermal testing is more sensitive than prick or puncture testing. For reactions to be equivalent, it takes about 1000-fold concentrate extract for skin prick testing.[1,3–5] Patch testing essentially uses the theory that a localized, confined, immune-mediated reaction to the extract can be elicited by introducing the agent transdermally. There continue to be ongoing studies about the efficacy of patch testing not only for allergy but also as the basis of evidence for diagnosing such conditions as anticonvulsant hypersensitivity syndrome.[6] The efficacy of patch testing versus other methods has also been studied in patients with nickel allergies.[7] **Table 1** shows a comparison between the commonly used percutaneous (prick puncture) method and the intradermal method of skin testing.

Skin Testing Devices

Although intradermal tests are performed using only a hypodermic needle and syringe, prick or puncture tests may be performed with a variety of devices. Some devices have a single stylus with several points, whereas others have multiple heads that allow up to ten tests to be performed at once.[3] The major concerns with the multihead devices involve the amount of trauma to the patient and issues with interpretation. Because of the variations in these devices, the proximity of the control to the allergen differs and there is a possibility of getting a false-positive result at the site of a negative control. In contrast, differences in application devices could produce a false-negative response.[3,8–10] Negative and positive controls are helpful in the interpretation of the allergen tests themselves, and are particularly important when using a multihead device.

Table 1
Comparison of intracutaneous (intradermal) and percutaneous route (prick or puncture) methods

Percutaneous Route (Prick or Puncture)	Intracutaneous Route (Intradermal)
Safer	More sensitive
Easy to administer	More reproducible
Rapid	Less specificity in testing
Little discomfort	Greater risks for systemic reactions (including fatalities)
Able to distinguish multiple allergies at one time	Useful in determining anaphylaxis, especially if caused by medication or venom
Steeper dose response curve	
Better correlates with clinical symptoms	Late-phase cutaneous responses are more likely to occur. This response is characterized by erythema, induration or edema, and dysesthesia
Preferred technique for IgE-mediated hypersensitivity	
Generally favored for initial screening due to fewer systemic reactions	

Prick or Puncture (Percutaneous) Method of Skin Testing

This test can be performed with a single test device or a multitest device. There is reported concern about the reproducibility of allergy skin test scoring and the interpretation when a single-prick device is used.[11,12] It is important for the nurse performing this test to be consistent with the amount of allergen placed on the device that is used to puncture the skin, at about a 90° angle. The puncture should be about 1 mm.[3] A positive control, which is usually a histamine, and a negative control, which is typically either saline or a 50% glycerinated human serum albumin saline, is applied at the same time as the allergens. It is a good idea to apply the negative control first.

Intradermal (Intracutaneous) Method of Skin Testing

These tests are commonly used by clinicians when the prick or puncture test yields negative results, yet the patient's clinical picture is suggestive of an allergy. This procedure is more sensitive, but less specific than the prick or puncture method.[1,13]

Intradermal tests are commonly used in the diagnosis of stings by insects such as wasps and bees, as well as for drug allergies. A recent study indicates that approximately 85% of allergists rely on the intradermal tests in patients who have negative test results when the skin prick test is negative, because of the sensitivity of the intradermal test.[14]

Intradermal tests should be performed with small volumes (approximately 0.02–0.05 mL) of allergens injected intracutaneously with a disposable 0.5- or 1.0-mL syringe. Although there are no clinical standards of exactly how much of the allergen should be used for testing, generally the starting dose of an intracutaneous allergen test ranges from 100- to 1000-fold more dilute than the allergen concentration used for prick or puncture tests.[1,3,15]

CONTROLS IN SKIN TESTING

Controls should be used with both forms of skin testing to assure accuracy of test results. A positive control is administered to assess the patient's responsiveness to histamine, which is responsible for immediate allergic responses. The negative control (typically saline or 50% glycerinated saline) should be applied before the antigen test to make sure that any wheals are the result of the antigen response and not a response to the glycerin used to preserve the antigen. The positive and negative controls should be administered using the same technique, which should be the same as that used to administer the antigen, or allergen.[16]

FACTORS THAT MAY AFFECT SKIN TEST REACTIVITY

There are numerous factors that may affect the reactivity of the skin test. The level of reactivity has implications for the interpretation of the test results. It is important for the nurse performing the skin test to know some of the possible confounding variables to reactivity of the test. Some of the common issues that impact results can derive from age,[17] medications,[3] and biologic rhythms such as menstruation.[18] **Table 2** provides an overview of many of these factors, with an explanation, and nursing considerations aimed at minimizing the influence of these factors on the interpretation of results.

ADVERSE REACTIONS TO ALLERGY SKIN TESTS

Immediate systemic reactions are more common with intradermal tests than with prick or puncture skin tests. Overall, very few fatalities have occurred with skin tests,

Table 2
Factors that influence skin test results

Factor	Explanation	Consideration
Age	Reactivity decreases with age, and peaks in late teens to early twenties, and then due to aging process, decreases over time. Histamine reactivity decreases more drastically at 50 and is thought to plateau around 60 years of age	Age is important for interpreting the timing of reactivity. Reactivity decreases with age, and peaks in late teens to early twenties, and then due to aging process, decreases. Also, for the elderly more prone to atrophic or photodamage, areas that are sun protected should be considered as sites for the test
Histamine sensitivity	Some people are born with more sensitive reactions to histamine. This can either increase or decrease the skin test reactivity	A thorough history and physical with connections to allergies, allergens, and any medications that might impact the skin test results is warranted
Location on the body	There are variants in test results based on where the test is performed. Variations are the result of sun damage to skin areas, and thickness of skin on different body areas. Differing results are thought to be the result of a greater number of capillaries in thicker skin and more opportunity for histamine release at the site	When testing, the same body area should be used. The size of the wheal should not be the only consideration. One must take into account the ratio between the histamine- and allergen-induced wheals Skin on forearm is less reactive than the skin on the back. Lower back skin is typically more reactive than upper back skin
Chronobiology	There is thought to be some circadian and circannual variability in individuals who impact skin testing	There is some opinion that circadian cycle within a 24-hour period might affect test results. There is no conclusive evidence to support this. Obvious circannual variations are most likely related to environmental allergens during specific times of the year
Menstrual cycle	During midcycle, reactions are larger than during menses	Important to note the stage of menstrual cycle in women of childbearing age

Medications	1. Histamine$_1$ antagonists suppress skin reaction to histamine and to the allergen 2. Tricyclic antidepressants have antihistamine properties 3. Glucocorticoids remain controversial, as there are conflicting studies about the length of use, and the effect on the test 4. Beta-blockers can increase reactivity	1. Omit Histamine$_1$ medications from the patient's regimen at least 24 hours before the test 2. There may be a delay in extract reaction, and the flare may last longer than normal 3. Note when a patient is on glucocorticoids, as the impact on the test is not well understood or documented 4. Note that patient is on a beta-blocker and that an increased reactivity is expected. In addition, beta-blockers can interfere with resuscitation efforts in the event of anaphylaxis or cardiac arrest
Disease processes	Different diseases processes may impact the reactivity of the test	The importance of a thorough history and physical is emphasized here. In cases of diseases such as cancer, the skin test reactivity might be suppressed. This can be the result of the disease process or the chemotherapy for the disease
Allergen extract quality	Weaker extracts may produce false-negative results	Like any medication, allergen extracts deteriorate over time. There is variation in potency over time based also on the type of extract. Extracts should be changed frequently, and close attention should be paid to expiration dates from the manufacturer
Proximity to positive control or other allergens	This is called the "bystander effect" in which an allergen extract is placed too close to a stronger positive extract resulting in a false-positive result	It is typically recommended that allergy skin tests be placed no closer than 5 cm apart. There have been some false-positive results reported with intradermal testing due to the "bystander effect"

Information to create this table was adapted from Refs. [1,3,9,17,18] but more have occurred with intradermal testing than with prick or puncture testing. Late-phase cutaneous responses are more likely to occur with intradermal testing than with percutaneous testing. This response is typically characterized by erythema, induration or edema, and dysesthesia.[15] Because of the potential for adverse reactions, as well as the desire to minimize the number unnecessary tests, the American Academy of Allergy, Asthma and Immunology and the American College of Allergy, Asthma and Immunology have jointly recommended that the number of skin tests and the allergens selected for testing should be based on the patient's age, history, environment, living conditions, occupation, and activities. Routine use of a large number of skin tests or routine annual skin testing without clinical indication is unjustifiable.[15]

About 80% of all adverse reactions are common and predictable, and are usually related to the activity of the allergen or, in cases of drug allergy testing, the actual pharmaceutics of the drug being tested. These reactions are usually referred to as "type A" reactions and are dose related, so can be controlled by eliminating the drug or titrating the amount of the drug.[19] Hypersensitivity reactions that are classified as "type B" reactions are less common, can be severe, and in some cases can be fatal. Such reactions are not predictable, are not dose dependent, and affect only predisposed individuals. "Type B" category reactions include such phenomena as drug intolerance, idiosyncratic reactions, and drug allergies.[19]

REPORTING SKIN TEST RESULTS

Because of the variability among clinicians, scoring on a qualitative scale (0–4+; positive or negative) is, for the most part, no longer used. There are recommendations, but there is no standard approach to reading the results; however, the report should include a quantitative measurement of the positive and negative control and the reactions to the different allergens in relation to the size of the positive and negative controls. Cox and colleagues[3] explain that in cases where a positive control has no reaction, the nonreacting allergens cannot be considered negative because of the possibility of a confounding factor affecting the allergen, leading to a false-negative interpretation. On the other hand, if a negative control has a positive reaction due to trauma caused by the device, or the proximity of the test to another test, the size of the negative control needs to be considered in relation to the interpretation of positive test results.

There are recent movements to make the measurement of the wheal more standard and precise with devices such as hand-held scanners and computer-assisted devices. The histamine control tests should be read 15 minutes after application at the peak of activity. The peak of allergen prick/puncture tests is usually 15 to 20 minutes after the application.[15] The current standard indicates that for a prick/puncture test, a response of at least 3 mm in diameter (with 10 mm erythema) more than the dilutant control done at the same time is evidence of the presence of allergen-specific IgE.[3,15] Measurements are typically done from end points of the longest diagonal.

Intracutaneous tests are read 10 to 15 minutes after injection. Histamine controls are typically read at 10 minutes, and allergen sites interpreted at 15 minutes after the injection. As with prick/puncture tests, the intradermal test results should include both the wheal and the amount of erythema, recorded in millimeters. Any wheal reaction larger than the negative control may indicate presence of specific IgE antibody. Because of the sensitivity of intracutaneous tests, small reactions that are positive may not be clinically significant.[15]

PATCH TESTING

Patch tests are thought to be most effective when the patient being tested has an unambiguous clinical presentation of contact allergy, and are tested with the chemical suspected of provoking the allergic response. Patch testing is used to define the causative agent in chronic eczematous dermatitis if an underlying allergic contact dermatitis is suspected. This test is of particular importance when one considers that there are more than 85,000 chemicals in the world today, and more than 3700 of these have been identified as contact allergens.[20,21]

There are 2 major variants of traditional patch tests, namely the atopy patch test and the repeated use test.[15] In a patch test, the allergen is usually placed on the patient's back with a device and remains there for 1 to 2 days, and the result is read after 1 day or 2 to 3 days. As there is no standard, this will vary among institutions and among clinicians within an institution. A photopatch test is a modification of the patch test when there is suspicion of a photoallergic or phototoxic reaction. In the photopatch test, after 1 day the patch is removed, and the area is exposed to UV light from 5 to 10 J/cm^2 UVA.[19] This test is read after 2, 3, and 4 days.

Because test reactivity is often diminished with UV exposure, patients who are undergoing patch tests should not have recent UV exposure from vacationing or sunbathing, working in the yard, or from tanning beds. A thorough review of the patient's medications should be completed, and the patient should not have any infectious diseases, fevers, or any active inflammatory processes (such as arthritis) at the time.[19]

Atopy patch tests for the diagnosis of a drug allergy are performed by incorporating liquid or powdered drugs into petroleum or aqueous solvents, which are added to a device called a "Finn Chamber." Atopy patch tests for food allergies are performed by adding dried or desiccated food mixed into aqueous solution, and applied to the back via a Finn Chamber.[15]

There are many limitations, due to lack of evidence, regarding patch testing. The role of patch testing in identifying clinical allergy to food is indeterminate.[15] The lack of standardization related to patch testing for the diagnosis of both food and drug allergy is a major limitation for this testing method.

SUMMARY

As with all laboratory tests, quality assurance standards should be met to ensure adequacy of the testing technique. It is recommended that persons performing skin tests undergo evaluation of their technique to improve the predictive values of skin testing, and to ameliorate the incidence or severity of adverse affects. It is important for the critical care nurse to understand the dynamics of the test and the possible risks, along with variables that can confound the results. By doing this, nurses will improve not only patient outcomes related to the testing itself but also the value and reliability of the most effective diagnostic tool available for allergic disease.

REFERENCES

1. Oppenheimer J, Nelson HS. Skin testing. Ann Allergy Asthma Immunol 2006; 96(Suppl 1):S6–12.
2. Blackley CH. Experimental researches on the causes and nature of catarrhus aestivus (hay fever or hay-asthma). England, London: Balliere Tindall & Cox; 1873.

3. Cox L, Williams B, Sicherer S, et al. Pearls and pitfalls of allergy diagnostic testing: Report from the American College of Allergy, Asthma, and Immunology/American Academy of Allergy, Asthma and Immunology Specific IgE Test Task Force. Ann Allergy Asthma Immunol 2008;101:580–92.

4. Gendo K, Larson EB. Evidence-based diagnostic strategies for evaluating suspected allergic rhinitis. Ann Intern Med 2004;140:278–89.

5. Indrajana T, Spieksma FT, Voorhorst R. Comparative study of the intracutaneous scratch and prick tests in allergy. Ann Allergy 1997;29:639–50.

6. Elzagallaai AA, Knowles SR, Rieder MJ, et al. Patch testing for the diagnosis of anticonvulsant hypersensitivity syndrome: a systematic review. Drug Saf 2009; 32(5):391–408.

7. Fischer LA, Johansen JD, Menne T. Nickel allergy: relationship between patch test and repeated open application test thresholds. Br J Dermatol 2007;157: 723–9.

8. Carr WW, Martin B, Howard RS, et al. Comparison of test devices for skin prick testing. J Allergy Clin Immunol 2005;116:341–6.

9. Nelson HS, Kolehmainen C, Lahr J, et al. A comparison of multiheaded devices for allergy skin testing. J Allergy Clin Immunol 2004;113:1218–9.

10. Newhall KK, Saltoun C. Skin testing in allergy. Ann Allergy Asthma Immunol 2004; 25(4 Suppl 1):S5–12.

11. McCann WA, Ownby DR. The reproducibility of the allergy skin test scoring and interpretation by board certified/board eligible allergists. Ann Allergy Asthma Immunol 2002;89:368–71.

12. Seshul M, Pilsbury H, Eby T. Use of intradermal dilutional testing and skin prick testing: clinical relevance and cost efficiency. Laryngoscope 2006;116:1530–8.

13. Wood RA, Phipatanakul W, Hamilton RG, et al. A comparison of skin prick tests, intradermal skin tests, and RASTs in the diagnosis of cat allergy. J Allergy Clin Immunol 1999;103:773–9.

14. Oppenheimer JJ, Nelson HS. Skin testing: a survey of allergists. Ann Allergy Asthma Immunol 2006;96:19–23.

15. Bernstein IL, Li JT, Bernstein DI. Allergy diagnostic testing: an updated practice parameter. Ann Allergy Asthma Immunol 2008;10:S1–148.

16. Krouse HJ. Diagnostic testing for inhalant allergies. ORL Head Neck Nurs 2007; 25(2):9–14.

17. King MJ, Lockey RF. Allergen prick-puncture skin testing in the elderly. Drugs Aging 2003;20(4):1011–7.

18. Kalogeromitros D, Katsarou A, Armenaka M, et al. Influence of the menstrual cycle on skin-prick test reactions to histamine, morphine and allergens. Clin Exp Allergy 1995;25:461–5.

19. Brockow K, Romano A. Skin tests in the diagnosis of drug hypersensitivity reactions. Curr Pharm Des 2008;14:2778–91.

20. Beltrani VS, Beltrani VP. Contact dermatitis. Ann Allergy Asthma Immunol 1997; 78(2):160–73.

21. Belsito DV. Patch testing with a standard allergen ("screening") tray: rewards and risks. Dermatol Ther 2004;17:231–9.

Ultrasound Studies

Melan Smith-Francis, MSN[a],*, Patty Orr, EdD[b]

KEYWORDS

• Ultrasound • Sonography • Abdominal ultrasound

There are a variety of ultrasound studies that the critical care nurse might encounter at the bedside, or in the outpatient clinic area. A thorough understanding of the process, what is expected, and the use of these tests enhances the nurse's role in caring for patients who are undergoing an ultrasound study, regardless of the specific setting.

OVERVIEW OF ULTRASOUND STUDIES

An ultrasound produces sound waves that are above the upper limit of the range for human hearing. These sound waves are used in medicine for diagnosis and treatment by allowing visualization inside the body through sound echoes that record structures beneath the skin. Reflection from different tissues allows a shadow picture to be recorded. Visualization of the interface of fluid-filled spaces and solid tissue is particularly accurate. Ultrasound technology creates images of internal organs and facilitates diagnoses and treatment of deep-tissue disorders. This testing uses a transducer or probe to project and receive the various sound wave signals as they pass into the body and reflect off of the solid organs. The transducer changes an electrical signal from the machine to ultrasound waves.[1] The transducer is connected to a computer with a display screen. Body tissues of different densities produce echoes, which are converted into electrical signals that are transformed into images of the body organs by the computer. The computer projects these images as interpreted by the variations of the echoes on the viewing screen.[2] A gel is first spread onto a person's skin to prevent distortion of the sound waves traveling through the skin. Enhanced Doppler technology can measure the movement of a substance, such as blood, in relation to the probe.

Although ultrasound is most commonly known for fetal monitoring during pregnancy, it is also often used for other organ system imaging because of its effectiveness in distinguishing variations of tissue structures without tissue radiation. Changes in physical symptoms or pain can indicate organ dysfunction, injury, or cancer; ultrasound testing can assist the physician in determining potential causes of the pain or

[a] School of Nursing, Austin Peay State University, McCord Building 312, PO Box 4658, Clarksville, TN 37044, USA
[b] School of Nursing, Austin Peay State University, McCord Building 305, PO Box 4658, Clarksville, TN 37044, USA
* Corresponding author.
E-mail address: smithfrancism@apsu.edu (M. Smith-Francis).

Crit Care Nurs Clin N Am 22 (2010) 83–93
doi:10.1016/j.ccell.2009.10.010
0899-5885/10/$ – see front matter © 2010 Elsevier Inc. All rights reserved.

physical symptoms. Ultrasound technology can also assist in visualization for guiding needle placement for biopsy or fluid drainage. Focused, high-frequency and high-intensity ultrasound can be used to destroy certain gallstones, calculi, and tumors. Soft-tissue musculoskeletal injuries, such as sprains and tears, can also benefit from high-intensity ultrasound. The high-intensity ultrasound promotes improved healing by vibrating the tissue and improving circulation at the involved site.

Specific clinical conditions can limit the effectiveness and quality of the test. Conditions limiting sound wave penetration include obesity, gas, or bone existing between the probe and target organ. Gas in the bowel, intestines, and stomach may prevent organ visualization behind the gas. Lungs filled with air impact the effectiveness of a chest ultrasound. Ultrasound effectiveness is also dependent upon the skill of the equipment operator and the quality of the equipment.

Four different modes of ultrasound imaging exist. A-mode uses a single transducer (device that converts acoustic waves to vibrations) to scan a line through the targeted part of the body with echoes measuring depth, size, and distances within the body structure. A-mode is used for calculi and tumor treatment with the destructive vibration caused by the sound waves. B-mode provides two-dimensional (2D) images by using many transducers in sequence. Heart motion study relies on M-mode, which uses a rapid sequence of B-mode scans whose images follow each other in sequence, to allow practitioners to see and measure motion range. The fourth mode of ultrasound is Doppler mode and is used to study the velocity of blood in veins and arteries. Doppler mode is often combined with B-mode scanning to measure blood flow and assess valve defects, hypertension, and arteriosclerosis. The term "duplex ultrasound" is used for vascular ultrasound and tests how blood moves through the arteries and veins. Images, processed by a computer from the transducer, are reflected on a screen and can be made into hard copy pictures.

Patients receiving an ultrasound test lie still on a table or bed and are allowed to talk to the person doing the test as the test is done. Preparation for the test depends on the area being scanned. For example, if the pelvis is being scanned, patients may be required to drink several glasses of water to have a full bladder. Fluids and food may be restricted for an abdominal scan. Patients will be nothing by mouth (NPO) after midnight if a biopsy is to occur. Patients are instructed to remove jewelry from the area of the body being scanned. The ultrasound examination usually takes between 30 and 60 minutes. After the study, patients can eat and return to normal activities. Activities may be restricted if a needle biopsy was performed. After a biopsy, patients should notify the physician if there is abnormal bleeding or swelling. Results from the ultrasound can be available within a few minutes to a few days.

Ultrasound testing is usually undertaken to detect if an abnormal structure (tumor, injury, calculi, lesion, and so forth) exists in the scanned body part. The test allows the examiner to have a view inside of the body to assist in making a diagnosis. The provider uses results of the test in addition to patients' signs and symptoms to make a diagnosis. As compared with CT scans, ultrasound is less expensive and faster for imaging purposes. Patients also avoid radiation exposure with the ultrasound test.[3]

Three-dimensional (3D) sonography is now an adjunct to standard 2-D sonography. Traditional 2D is very operator dependent for a quality examination and is more time intensive, whereas 3D does not require an operator during the procedure and takes about half of the time to administer.[3] The probe is placed over the body part and is not moved. The needed views are manipulated to create the 3-D image that is very detailed.[1] This newer cross-sectional method of sonography provides the ability to reconstruct any plane with improved image quality compared with other cross-sectional modalities, such as CT.[3]

Ultrasound waves are considered safe with no known side effects. Sonograms have been used in pregnancy for more than 40 years with no reports of side effects for either the woman or fetus. The Doppler device used in fetal monitoring, using low-intensity ultrasound, does not produce any adverse heating effects. Doppler instrumentation for arterial studies uses higher intensity of sound, producing some heat in the tissues, and is not considered appropriate for fetal monitoring.[1] The scans are usually painless. There are no known side effects, such as bleeding, reaction to chemicals, or infections as may occur with other diagnostic testing. Medications do not interfere with the testing.[4] Ultrasound testing findings may relate abnormal findings or indicate the need for further testing. The nurse must be sensitive to patients' anxiety and offer support in coping with any distressing news.

Ultrasound studies are used to assess, screen, diagnose, and assist treatment for many organ systems. Applicable tests for specific systems include testing for obstetrics, gynecology and other abdominal structures, breasts, cardiac, blood vessels, thyroid gland, and certain joints. Elias and Semelka (2006)[5] urge providers to consider variables, such as image quality, consistent display of normal and diseased anatomy, availability, cost, comfort, and safety before choosing ultrasound as a diagnostic tool.

ABDOMINAL AND RETROPERITONEUM ULTRASOUND TESTING

An abdominal and retroperitoneum examination may include the entire area or may single out a single organ, or several organs, or may focus on a certain body function, such as the biliary system. Common indications for the abdominal ultrasound include pain, hematuria, jaundice, presence of a mass or organomegaly, abnormal lab findings suggesting abdominal pathology, metastatic disease or primary neoplasm, abdominal trauma, and planning for an invasive procedure. Testing analyzes the abdomen for free fluid of the peritoneum and can assess each of the following organs: liver, gallbladder and biliary tract, pancreas, spleen, bowel, and abdominal wall.[6] Contrast materials in the intestine can impede the visualization of internal organs, and as a result abdominal ultrasound should be completed before diagnostic testing that requires contrast material.[7] The retroperitoneum study can assess the kidneys, bladder, adrenal glands, aorta, and inferior vena cava.[6]

TRANSVAGINAL ULTRASOUND
Case Report

YH, a 62-year-old postmenopausal Caucasian woman, called her primary gynecologist to complain of intermittent bleeding. After further inquiry it was determined that she denied pain and sustained uterine polyps were removed 1 year prior because of postmenopausal spotting. She was advised to make an appointment to evaluate the status of her uterine lining by pelvis and transvaginal ultrasound. The radiologist read the report and forwarded the following to the primary gynecologist: slightly enlarged uterus in normal position, which measures $11.5 \times 3.6 \times 5.6$ cm in size. The endometrium measures 0.8 cm in thickness. There were no uterine masses or other significant abnormality. Bilateral ovaries were unremarkable in size, configuration, and echotexture. There was no adnexal or pelvic mass or abnormal collection of fluid. It was concluded that there was evidence of an enlarged uterus. YH's second follow-up ultrasound revealed the following: the uterus measures $11 \times 2.9 \times 5.7$ cm in dimension, which was similar to the measurement noted on the previous study. The endometrial strip was somewhat thickened, measuring 7.2 mm in thickness. Previous measurement was 8.3 mm. It was concluded that there was an enlarged uterus with thickened endometrium. The appearance was similar to that noted on the previous study.

YH's initial evaluation included a history, physical examination, and an endometrial ultrasound. This case represents the usefulness of ultrasound to identify bleeding in the postmenopausal woman. YH was presenting with one of the primary indications for pelvic ultrasound. The transvaginal ultrasound will produce a quality image and has a high index of diagnostic confidence and will therefore be sufficient evidence to treat YH based on this diagnostic tool alone.[5] Other diagnostic tools to evaluate her case may be an endometrial biopsy as well as CT or MRI. To rule out evidence of a neoplasm, the transvaginal ultrasound must indicate a thickened endometrium. This minimally invasive assessment will afford the radiologist, and practitioner, the ability to assess the status of neoplasms that may be present. This transvaginal ultrasound assessment is specific for YH in that it will identify the cause of the irregular vaginal bleeding. Using this specific tool will save YH time, money, and exposure to unnecessary interventions.[8] To improve the diagnosis and treatment of endometrial cancer, further research for endometrial cancer will include 3-D ultrasound.[9]

The transvaginal ultrasound is an imaging technique used to visualize the genital tract in women. The Doppler is inserted directly into the vagina close to the pelvic structures. Although the transvaginal method provides a view of a smaller area, the images are often clearer and less distorted than what can be obtained through transabdominal ultrasound technology. Indications for using the transvaginal ultrasound include testing of the endometrium for abnormal bleeding or fertility problems. It is also indicated for assessing pain, congenital malformations of the ovaries and uterus, ovarian cysts and tumors, pelvic infections, bladder abnormalities, a misplaced intrauterine device, and infertility.

Preparation for the transvaginal ultrasound includes not drinking liquids for 4 hours before the test. Patients lie on their backs with the hips raised and are asked to lie still as the transducer is moved to adjust for certain views. Patients are taught to assess for signs of infection or bleeding if a biopsy was done during the testing.[10]

A combination of transvaginal and abdominal ultrasound is recommended to optimally assess the ovaries for early signs of ovarian cancer because the location of the ovaries varies in each woman. Because each test gives different views, it is recommended that both tests are used to detect any signs of early ovarian cancer.[11] Carriers of BRCA1 or BRCA2 genes, which indicate increased genetic prediction for hereditary breast or ovarian cancer, are often encouraged to have regular surveillance of the ovaries with ovarian ultrasounds and ultrasound of the breast. Claes reported literature findings that demonstrated that 59% to 73% of carriers had high use of ovarian ultrasound screening when positive for BRCA1 or BRCA2 and 87% to 93% had high use of mammography. A CT scan may also be recommended for the abdomen and pelvis area if ovarian cancer is suspected.[12]

TRAUMA

The clinical guidelines for use of ultrasound in trauma patients were developed collaboratively by the American College of Emergency Physicians and the American Institute of Ultrasound Medicine (AIUM). The specific guideline is a focused assessment with sonography for trauma (FAST).[13] The FAST examination is an assessment that lasts less than 5 minutes. It uses reference points or windows within the abdomen to distinguish any free fluid from the solid organ masses. The reference points are inclusive of pericardial, perihepatic, perisplenic and pelvic region.[14] The most common organ used as a reference point in trauma is the perihepatic region. Upon assessment, the sonographer will identify fluid versus organ, which is differentiated by shadows of gray to black.[15] The fluid will most often be black and take the shape of the container it is in.[14] The guidelines for testing maximize the detection of free fluid. Because hemorrhage into the abdomen and chest is often covert, clinical detection can be difficult. Trauma patients may not show symptoms, such as decreased blood pressure and tachycardia, until 30% of blood volume is lost. Ultrasound, used for the detection of hemorrhage in the peritoneum, has a sensitivity of approximately 90%.[16] Ultrasound equipment is portable, does not impede the trauma team, and can be used at the bedside. The FAST testing can often take the place of more invasive surgical procedures for evaluation purposes.

Training of the trauma surgeons and emergency physicians is critical to obtain a fast and accurate interpretation of the ultrasound in the emergency setting. Those patients positive for fluid in the peritoneum and pleural cavities or are physiologically unstable require immediate surgery. Stable patients with suspicion for increased fluid may benefit from repeating a previous negative scan. Studies have shown benefit of serial ultrasounds as part of a follow-up for detecting free fluid after patients are presented with blunt abdominal trauma.[17]

Although there are no contraindications for doing the FAST examination, there are limitations. Jones and Blavias identify body characteristics, injury location, history of prior surgeries, presence of clotted blood, patient position, and the amount of fluid present as limitations to the FAST examination. The rationales for these limitations range from the simple sound speed of the transducer to the pressure gradients of fluid, the position of the client, and gravity. However, a fluid-filled bladder facilitates the visualization of free fluid in the pelvis. Because free fluid concentrates to the dependent part of the pelvis, free fluid can be missed if patients have an empty bladder. It is very important to do the sonography before a Foley catheter is inserted. In the trauma room ultrasound is a valuable tool in establishing which patients are likely to benefit from early surgery for fluid accumulation in the peritoneum and pleural cavities. The specific site of injury can be localized by the sonography.[13]

In the majority of the studies examined, the accuracy of sonographic specificity is 90% or greater.[17] However, there are other areas of concern regarding the FAST examination. The FAST examination might miss correctable injuries. For this reason, it is recommended to use sonography only as the initial examination, and later perform a CT scan, particularly for hemodynamically stable people or those with an intra-abdominal injury. There were a small amount of studies that suggested serial sonography as a follow-up examination to distinguish free fluid in those with blunt abdominal trauma because if there is active bleeding the amount of free fluid will increase over time. McGahan and colleagues[17] suggest studying the effectiveness of using FAST to identify solid-organ injuries and to diagnose pneumothoraces by identifying the absence of the sliding lung.

Freeman (1999) mentions the debate between using diagnostic peritoneal lavage (DPL) or ultrasounds on unstable trauma patients. DPL is what has usually been used in the past. During this procedure an incision is placed in the abdomen for a blunt catheter. A liter of warm, sterile isotonic fluid is put into the peritoneal cavity and drained. Blood, white cells, or bacteria would indicate an intra-abdominal injury. This procedure is invasive and takes up to 20 minutes and cannot be repeated. On the other hand, ultrasounds can be very quick and noninvasive. Training for ultrasounds is basic. Small amounts of intraperitoneal blood might not be detected; however, it depends on the experience of the operator. In addition, ultrasound is considered safe. Heller refers to the official position of the AIUM which validates that no confirmed biologic effects on patients or instrument operators caused an exposure at intensities typical of present diagnostic ultrasound instruments have ever been reported.[15] Although the possibility exists that such biologic effects may be identified in the future, current data indicates that the benefits of the prudent use of diagnostic ultrasound outweigh the risks, if any, that may be present.

McGahan and colleagues (2002) also support the use of ultrasounds for trauma scan. They have also found instances that ultrasounds were used to evaluate thoracic abnormalities in patients with pleural effusions, pneumothoraces, and pericardial effusions.[17] An ultrasound can also be used to determine whether patients have an abdominal aortic aneurysm. Abdominal aortic aneurysm screens should be used for male patients more than 65 years old, female patients more than 65 years old with any cardiovascular risks, and those with a family history of aneurismal disease. If patients present with, but not limited to, any obvious abdominal mass, back or abdominal pain, or any known aneurysm disease, an abdominal aorta ultrasound would be warranted.[18] Other uses for the emergency use of ultrasonography include ultrasound-guided procedures, such as venous cannulation, lumbar puncture, pericardiocentesis, paracentesis, thoracentesis, abscess drainage, pacemaker insertion/capture confirmation, foreign body localization/removal, and fracture reduction.[14]

The American College of Emergency Physicians supports application of this technology and encourages appropriate training and credentialing through an ultrasonography curriculum.[15] Training is required to interpret the images. There are three levels of training for ultrasounds. The first level is a basic overview of the use of ultrasounds and is only a 2-day (16 hour) workshop. The second level requires a period of supervision involving 150 mentored scans and also a 16-hour lecture and practical course. The third level involves advance practice to achieve the Diploma in Diagnostic Ultrasound. Most clinicians require at least a level two training.[16]

OBSTETRIC
Case Report

MF, a 35-year-old African American woman, gravida 1, para 1, 12-weeks gestation called the midwifery clinic after hours to report spotting. After further inquiry it was determined that MF experienced spotting during the night while waking to use the restroom. She denied cramping and said that the spotting progressively improved throughout the night. She was encouraged to present to the office the following business day to have an ultrasound. The next day, a limited ultrasound was performed to reveal that within the uterus was a well-defined gestational sac. A fetus was clearly delineated. Cardiac activity was seen on real-time examination. There was a small retrochorionic hemorrhage seen at the inferior margin of the placenta. The sonogram confirmed an intrauterine pregnancy with normal progression since the prior study. There was a marginal hemorrhage measuring $30 \times 25 \times 18$ mm. The report was read by the radiologist, which was then forwarded to the primary midwife.

This case represents the ultrasounds' usefulness in screening for first trimester bleeding in pregnancy. MF was experiencing what at least 25% of women experience in their first trimester of pregnancy.[19] Although MF had a primary ultrasound to identify early gestational development, this occurrence calls for a repeat transvaginal ultrasound. Evaluation and management is based on MF's gestational age and the clinical findings listed above. Therefore, the primary assessment tool should be the transvaginal as opposed to transabdominal. Jauniaux and colleagues (2005)[20] mention that understanding the pitfalls of normal-pregnancy ultrasonography will assist the provider with the diagnostic assessment and management of high-risk pregnancies. The transvaginal ultrasound should detect the gestational sac and the placental function, which will give the radiologist a good understanding of the status of the pregnancy. The best predictor of pregnancy outcomes stems from using the transvaginal ultrasound after 7-weeks gestational age.[19] Ultrasound techniques have revolutionized the obstetric realm of predicting maternal fetal outcomes. It has become a safe, noninvasive, economical assessment imaging tool to use for normal and high-risk pregnancies.

A very common use of ultrasound testing is in obstetrics when ultrasound is used for assessing the progression of pregnancy. Fetal ultrasound uses the lowest possible ultrasonic exposure settings for diagnostic purposes when there is valid medical reason. Scanning can be performed either transabdominal or transvaginally. Obstetric guidelines developed by the American College of Obstetrics and Gynecology (ACOG) and AIUM do not support the use of routine sonography screening for all pregnant women.[21] Based upon the guideline from the AIUM and ACOG an obstetric ultrasound may be indicated once during the first trimester and during the second or third trimester. Indications during the first trimester are to confirm the presence of an intrauterine pregnancy and to estimate the gestational age. The uterus and cervix are evaluated for the presence of a gestational sac with a yolk sac or embryo. The crown-rump length is recorded, if possible, to best determine the gestational age. Indications for an ultrasound during the first trimester can also be to assess for possible maternal and fetal abnormalities. Ectopic pregnancy, vaginal bleeding, pelvic pain, multiple gestations, and pelvic masses are potential maternal abnormalities that could be indications for the ultrasound. Fetal anomalies could include assessment for cardiac deficits, anencephaly in high-risk patients, or other congenital diseases.

Indications for second and third trimester ultrasounds, in addition to the reasons given previously for the first trimester ultrasound, include: adjunct to amniocentesis, suspected fetal death, evaluation of fetal well-being, suspected placental abruption, premature rupture of membranes, and evaluation of placenta location. A standard ultrasonic fetal examination includes fetal cardiac activity, fetal number and presentation, and estimate of fluid volume. Fetal head, femur, and abdominal measurements are assessed and a fetal weight is estimated. Gestational age is also assessed.[22]

A fetal sonographic examination is done during the first and third trimester. During the examination the fetal presentation, amount of amniotic fluid, cardiac activity, placental position, biometry, and an anatomic survey is determined. Fetal ultrasounds should only be done when there is a valid reason and a limited ultrasound should be done when there is an area of concern.[21]

A high-risk pregnancy occurs in women with past medical history, such as diabetes or epilepsy. A Doppler ultrasound is used in the majority of all medical fields. A Doppler ultrasound works by measuring how the direction and velocity of blood flow affects sound waves. It can be measured from the umbilical artery, middle cerebral artery, ductus venous, and uterine arteries. Doppler sonography is one of the best ways to monitor a high-risk pregnancy because it is noninvasive and can be conducted in a short amount of time. There is some question whether a 3-D ultrasound is more helpful to doctors and patients. Three-dimensional ultrasounds improve the evaluation of organ circulation. It is also helpful in showing centralization of fetal circulation, deducing that it is possible that 3-D ultrasounds increase the chance of finding fetal anomalies. Blincoe found studies that reported more congenital anomalies in high-risk pregnancies; however, detection was worse compared with low-risk pregnancies. Ultrasounds are an effective way to monitor pregnancies for irregularities.[23]

Filly and Crane (2002) were concerned with the debate about who should receive sonography and when. According to the National Institute of Health (NIH), if a pregnant woman is young, healthy, begins seeing her obstetrician early, and has no serious medical history for her and her family then she does not need a sonography. In 1984, the NIH panel stated that there was no evidence to warrant sonographic screening in low-risk pregnancies.[22]

Diagnostic ultrasound is considered safe for the fetus during pregnancy. The procedure should use the lowest possible exposure setting to gain the diagnostic information and should be performed only for a valid medical indication. Use of ultrasound without a physician's order may be in violation of state laws. To prevent nonmedical use of ultrasounds and potential dangers to the fetus, several state legislatures have introduced legislation to regulate ultrasound ownership and use.[24]

BREAST
Case Report

LC, a 22-year-old Caucasian woman presented for a yearly physical. She complained of a right upper quadrant breast lump. Her past medical, surgical, and gynecologic history was remarkable. She denied any pain or alteration in breast tissue. She noticed the lump several months before her visit. Her breast examination was within normal limits with the exception of a 2-cm, tender, palpable mass in the upper left-breast quadrant. She was advised to follow up with a mammogram. Shortly thereafter the provider called her back into the office to request she follow up with an ultrasound to rule out a solid or fluid-filled cyst.

LC's case represents a common complaint for women of all age groups. Based on her age in conjunction with the density of her breast, she was a good candidate to screen with an ultrasound as opposed to a mammogram.[5,25] Bond (2008) acknowledges that using mammography is up to 50% less sensitive in women with dense breast tissue and therefore not perfect in detecting disease. Using an ultrasound to evaluate the breasts is usually used strictly to differentiate between cystic and solid lesions. Therefore, not only will ultrasound prove beneficial to her based on its sensitivity but it is more economical and has improved treatment outcomes.[26]

Breast ultrasounds are used primarily to investigate a specific problem area of the breast. A palpable lump or a mass discovered by mammography is often further evaluated by ultrasound. The ultrasound is helpful in distinguishing between a solid mass and a fluid-filled cyst. Breast ultrasound is particularly effective in women less than 35 years old whose mammograms are difficult to interpret because of the high density of the breast tissue. The guidance of a needle for biopsy of breast tissue is often aided by ultrasound, and patients often report less discomfort compared with a surgical biopsy. Lack of radiation makes ultrasounds ideal for patients who are pregnant when breast abnormalities exist. Breast ultrasound imaging is complementary to mammography by providing data in a tomographic format. A palpable cancer is much less likely to be obscured by overlying parenchyma with breast ultrasound.[27]

A breast ultrasound is used to determine whether there are palpable masses in women less than 30 years old or those that are lactating. It is used in addition to other testing methods to check abnormalities. Ultrasound of the breast can also be used for those who are experiencing problems with implants or as a treatment plan for therapy.[28]

Durfee and colleagues (2000) implemented a study to discover the effectiveness of sonography in detecting breast cancer. They are adamant when stating that ultrasound should be used in conjunction with mammography because both techniques give different forms of data. From their experiment, they found that 99% of cancers were visible when they used ultrasound and mammography.[27]

TRANSTHORACIC ECHOCARDIOGRAM

The transthoracic echocardiogram (TTE) is used to detect cardiac valvular defects, such as mitral valvular prolapse. The diameters of the heart chambers, atrial septal defects, patent ductus arteriosus, and pleural effusion are often diagnosed with an echocardiogram. Cross-sectional echocardiograms can detect changes in coronary vessels and the blood flow through the vessels. With Doppler echocardiography it is possible to localize and determine the amount of obstruction in the cardiovascular system.[29] Doppler flow velocity integrals provides flow volume information, such as left-ventricular systolic function (ejection fraction), regional wall motion, left-ventricular filling pressure, and left-ventricular diastolic function.[29]

Patients having a TTE experience little if any pain and no radiation exposure. TTE stress tests performed with exercise or vasoactive medication, such as dobutamine, involves minimal risk of arrhythmia, ischemia, or hypertension.[29] Continuous monitoring of electrocardiograms, heart rate, and blood pressure must be performed during the stress testing. Patients should be NPO before stress testing echocardiography.[7]

THYROID

An ultrasound can be used for aspiration or biopsy of any irregularities of the thyroid or any masses on the neck. An ultrasound for the thyroid can be used as a follow-up procedure from other imaging examinations; it determines the presence, size, and location of the thyroid gland, it is used on patients who have a chance of developing occult thyroid malignancy, to check up on current diseases, and to locate any abnormalities.[30]

MUSCULOSKELETAL

An ultrasound can be used for a full assessment of a joint. The shoulder, elbow, wrist, hand, hip, knee, ankle, foot, nerves, and tissue mass can be evaluated. An ultrasound can also be used to determine whether foreign bodies are in soft tissue. For an interventional musculoskeletal ultrasound cysts, fluid collections, abscesses, biopsy, injections, and foreign-body retrieval can be done. An ultrasound provides visualization of needles and shows the pathway for insertion.[31]

ARTERIES

Ultrasounds can be used to determine any injuries of the extremity arteries. Injuries will be investigated if patients have limb pain, ulceration, gangrene, rest pain, wound healing, cold sensitivity or discoloration, possible thoracic outlet syndrome, possible graft, arterial harvesting, and also for follow-ups and surveillance. Arterial occlusive disease can also be detected with an ultrasound. A peripheral venous ultrasound is used to determine whether patients have an obstruction, insufficiency, grafts, thrombosis, and also for follow-ups. The ankle-brachial index, a ratio of the pressure in the legs and arms, is a test to evaluate peripheral vascular disease. A handheld Doppler identifies the dorsalis pedis artery and posterior pedal pulses in the ankles. A sphygmomanometer is inflated to measure the pressure in the ankle. The ankle-brachial index is calculated by dividing the highest pressure in each ankle by the higher systolic pressure. An index between 0.9 and 1.3 represents a normal value.[32]

SUMMARY

This article focuses on the clinical use of ultrasound with obstetric, gynecologic, and trauma patients by reviewing recent case studies of the use of ultrasound for diagnostic purposes. This article also summarizes the AIUM guidelines for use in several types of patients. The AIUM is a multidisciplinary association whose purpose is to "advance the art and science of ultrasound in medicine and research through educational, scientific, literary, and professional activities."[33] The organization provides guidelines, in conjunction with many professional organizations, such as the American College of Cardiology and American College of Obstetrics and Gynecology. AIUM also serves as an accrediting body for ultrasound practices.

REFERENCES

1. Corbett J. Laboratory tests and diagnostic procedures with nursing diagnoses. 7th edition. New Jersey (NJ): Prentice Hall; 2008.
2. Urden L, Stacy K, Lough M, editors. Critical care nursing: diagnosis and management. St Louis (MO): Mosby Inc; 2002. p. 803.
3. Benacerraf B, Shipp T, Bromley B. How sonographic tomography will change the face of obstetric sonography: a pilot study. J Ultrasound Med 2005;24:371–8.
4. Cooper P. Ultrasound scanning. Clinical Reference Systems 2008.
5. Elias J, Semelka R. Utility of ultrasound in the modern imaging paradigm. 2006. Medscape CME. Available at: http://www.cme.medscape.com. Accessed April 6, 2009.
6. Practice guideline for the performance of an ultrasound examination of the abdomen and/or retroperitoneum. American Institute of Ultrasound in Medicine. Available at: http://www.aium.org. Accessed March 24, 2009.
7. Craig M. Essentials of sonography and patient care. 2nd edition. St Louis (MO): Elsevier; 1993.
8. McFarlin B. Ultrasound assessment of the endometrium for irregular vaginal bleeding. J Midwifery Womens Health 2006;51:440–9.
9. Graebe R. The role of imaging techniques in gynecology. In: DeCherney A, Nathan L, editors. Current obstetric & gynecologic diagnosis & treatment. 9th edition. Ohio (OH): McGraw-Hill Medical: 2002. p. 57–64.
10. Sims J. Transvaginal ultrasound. In: Jacqueline LL, editor. The gale encyclopedia of medicine. 3rd edition. Detroit: Gale; 2006.
11. Martin V. Straight talk about ovarian cancer: learn how to help patients recognize and defeat this insidious malignancy. Nursing 2005;35:36–41.
12. Claes E, Evers-Kiebooms G, Decryenaere M, et al. Surveillance behavior and prophylactic surgery after predictive testing for hereditary breast/ovarian cancer. Behav Med 2005;31:93–105.
13. Practice guideline for the performance of the focused assessment with sonography for trauma examination. American Institute of Ultrasound in Medicine. Available at: http://www.aium.org. Accessed March 24, 2009.
14. Jones R, Blaivas M. The handbook of ultrasound in trauma and critical illness. Ohio (OH): American College of Emergency Physicians; 2003.
15. Heller M, Dietrich J. Ultrasound in emergency medicine. Pennsylvania: W.B. Saunders Company; 1995.
16. Freeman P. The role of ultrasound in the assessment of the trauma patient. Aust J Rural Health 1999;7:85–9.
17. McGahan J, Richards J, Gillen M. The focused abdominal sonography for trauma scan: pearls and pitfalls. J Ultrasound Med 2002;21:789–800.
18. Practice guideline for the performance of diagnostic and screening ultrasound examinations of the abdominal aorta. American Institute of Ultrasound in Medicine. Available at: http://www.aium.org. Accessed March 24, 2009.

19. Thorstensen K. Midwifery management of first trimester bleeding and early pregnancy loss. J Midwifery Womens Health 2000;45(6):481–97.
20. Jauniaux E, Johns J, Burton G. The role of ultrasound imaging in diagnosing and investigating early pregnancy failure. Ultrasound Obstet Gynecol 2005;25: 613–24.
21. Practice guideline for the performance of obstetric ultrasound examinations. American Institute of Ultrasound in Medicine. Available at: http://www.aium.org. Accessed March 24, 2009.
22. Filly R, Crane J. Routine obstetric sonography. J Ultrasound Med 2002;21:713–8.
23. Blincoe A. Doppler sonography: improving outcome in high risk pregnancy. Br J Midwifery 2007;15:650–3.
24. Uhles J. Unsound ultrasounds? An examination of state legislature regulating non-medical ultrasound use and private ownership. J Leg Med 2007;28:263–82.
25. Zonderland H. The role of ultrasound in the diagnosis of breast cancer. Semin Ultrasound CT MR 2000;21:317–24.
26. S. Bond Combined screening with ultrasound and mammography vs. mammography alone in women at elevated risk of breast cancer. (Review of Screening with ultrasound at the time of mammography improves disease detection in women at higher risk for breast cancer, but false positives increase). JAMA 2008;299:2151–63.
27. Durfee SM, Selland DG, Smith DN, et al. Sonographic evaluation of clinically palpable breast cancers invisible on mammography. Breast J 2000;6:247–51.
28. Practice guideline for the performance of a breast ultrasound examination. American Institute of Ultrasound in Medicine. Available at: http://www.aium.org. Accessed March 24, 2009.
29. Cheitlin M, Alpert J, Armstrong W, et al. ACC/AHA practice guidelines. The American College of Cardiology. Available at: http://www.acc.org. Accessed April 6, 2009.
30. Practice guideline for the performance of a thyroid and parathyroid ultrasound examination. American Institute of Ultrasound in Medicine. Available at: http://www.aium.org. Accessed March 24, 2009.
31. Practice guideline for the performance of the musculoskeletal ultrasound examination. American Institute of Ultrasound in Medicine. Available at: http://www.aium.org. Accessed March 24, 2009.
32. Practice guideline for the performance of a physiologic evaluation of extremity arteries. American Institute of Ultrasound in Medicine. Available at: http://www.aium.org. Accessed March 24, 2009.
33. American Institute of Ultrasound in Medicine. Mission Statement & Constitution/ Bylaws. Available at: http://www.aium.org/aboutAIUM/constitution.aspx. Accessed March 23, 2009.

Centesis Studies in Critical Care

Cathy A. Cooper, EdD, MSN, RN, CNE

KEYWORDS

- Amniocentesis • Arthrocentesis • Paracentesis
- Pericardiocentesis • Thorocentesis

Critical care nurses have a vital role in caring for clients undergoing centesis studies. The word "centesis" means to perforate, puncture, or tap as with a needle.[1] It is the act of puncturing a body cavity, joint, organ, or space with a hollow needle to draw out fluid.[2] All centesis studies are invasive procedures, which are typically performed for either therapeutic or diagnostic purposes. On occasion, medications may also be administered during a centesis procedure.

CENTESIS STUDIES IN GENERAL

The following guidelines broadly apply to all centesis studies; however, health care organizations and agencies may have variant procedures for nurses who are assisting with a centesis. It is important for the nurses to know the policies and guidelines that have been adopted by their employing institution. Additionally, if the client receives sedation during a centesis procedure one should follow the agency's protocol for documentation and monitoring procedural sedation. Typically, the scope of nursing responsibilities includes (1) educating the client and family about the procedure; (2) preparing the client and environment for the procedure; (3) assessing and documenting the client's status before, during, and after the procedure; and (4) assisting the health care provider performing the centesis as needed.

As with any procedure, it is essential to establish positive patient identification, and verify that the client has given informed consent. This is typically done by having them sign a consent form before the procedure. Check for allergies, especially to skin antiseptics or local anesthetic, and report any medication allergies to the health care provider performing the procedure. Note and report any abnormal laboratories (ie, partial thromboplastin time, international normalized ratio, platelet count), and remember to verify the correct site for the procedure that is about to be performed. The client should have an empty bladder with the exception of an amniocentesis. It is important to verify that the client understands the need for the procedure, what to expect during the procedure, and what is expected during and following the

School of Nursing, Middle Tennessee State University, 1500 Greenland Drive, PO Box 81, Murfreesboro, TN 37132, USA
E-mail address: cacooper@mtsu.edu

Crit Care Nurs Clin N Am 22 (2010) 95–108
doi:10.1016/j.ccell.2009.10.003
0899-5885/10/$ – see front matter © 2010 Elsevier Inc. All rights reserved.

ccnursing.theclinics.com

procedure. Reassure the client that the health care team will remain vigilant during the procedure, and that they will tend to any need the client may have during the procedure.

The health care provider reviews specific risks and possible complications as they relate to the client's individual circumstances. A major contraindication for centesis studies includes clients who are unable to follow directions or cooperate during the procedure, or clients with an uncorrected coagulopathy.

Explain that their health care provider cleans the appropriate anatomic area with an antiseptic solution, drapes it, and injects a local anesthetic before inserting the needle. Inform your client that they may experience a burning sensation from the anesthetic, and feel some pressure at the site when the needle is introduced. Emphasize the importance of remaining still during the procedure because any sudden movement could dislodge the needle. Fluid samples obtained during the centesis procedure are sent to the laboratory for analysis. Often the nurse is responsible for labeling or numbering the tubes. Following removal of the needle, a small bandage is applied to the puncture site.

Documentation should include the type of centesis procedure performed and by whom. Additionally, documentation should include color and amount of any fluid obtained; the number of specimens or tubes sent for analysis; the laboratory tests to be performed; how the client tolerated the procedure, including vital signs; any complications; all medications administered including dosage, route, and time; and an assessment of the puncture site postprocedure.

Because there are a variety of centesis procedures that the critical care nurse might encounter, the following centesis procedures are discussed more in depth: amniocentesis, arthrocentesis, lumbar puncture, paracentesis, pericardiocentesis, and thoracentesis. By becoming more familiar with each of these procedures, the critical care nurse gains confidence in caring for clients when these procedures are indicated.

AMNIOCENTESIS

Other than in critical care obstetric units, critical care nurses may encounter pregnant clients following trauma, or in cases where the client is experiencing comorbidity at which time an amniocentesis may be indicated. Amniotic fluid is the fluid that surrounds and protects the fetus during pregnancy. Enclosed in a sac within the uterus, amniotic fluid contains fetal cells and a number of proteins and hormones (ie, alpha fetoprotein) that are produced by the fetus. Under usual conditions, amniocentesis is performed in an outpatient setting or a health care provider's office. Early amniocentesis (done between 11 and 14 weeks after the last menstrual period) is not typically recommended because it poses a higher risk of miscarriage and other complications than a second trimester amniocentesis.[3] Amniocentesis is most commonly done in the second trimester between 15 and 20 weeks of pregnancy. After the fifteenth week of pregnancy, the two layers of fetal membranes have usually fused sufficiently to safely allow withdrawal of a sample of amniotic fluid. Amniocentesis, as a diagnostic procedure, is performed for different reasons and during different trimesters of pregnancy, including diagnosing or ruling out certain birth defects and genetic disorders (genetic amniocentesis), and establishing the level of lung maturity in anticipation of delivery (maturity amniocentesis).[4]

Genetic Amniocentesis

Genetic amniocentesis is offered to a client if the results may significantly impact management of the pregnancy, including continuation or termination. Genetic amniocentesis may be recommended as follow-up to an abnormal prenatal screening test, a previous pregnancy with a chromosomal abnormality or neural tube defect, if the client's age is 35 or older, or in cases where there is a family history of a specific genetic disorder. Very rarely is a genetic amniocentesis done as early as the eleventh week of pregnancy.[5]

Maturity Amniocentesis

The purpose of a maturity amniocentesis is to determine the extent to which the fetus' lungs are mature enough for delivery. This type of amniocentesis is suggested if an early delivery is being considered and in association with preventing a pregnancy complication. It is usually performed between 32 and 39 weeks of gestation. Amniocentesis at this stage poses minimal risks to the woman and fetus, and can offer assurance that the fetus is ready for delivery. Several recent studies, however, suggest that testing for fetal lung maturity at the more advanced gestational age (>36 weeks) is neither reliable nor cost effective, and might be best reserved for fetuses between 32 and 36 weeks gestation.[6]

Amniocentesis can also be performed in the third trimester to diagnose uterine or fetal infections, or help evaluate the severity of anemia in fetuses with Rh disease. Information from the amniocentesis helps the health care provider determine whether a fetus may require a blood transfusion. Rarely is amniocentesis used to decrease the volume of amniotic fluid.

Risks Associated with Amniocentesis

The nurse caring for a woman undergoing an amniocentesis and the client who is going to have an amniocentesis should be aware of the risks associated with amniocentesis. These risks include the following.

Miscarriage
The risk of miscarriage is highest when the procedure is done early in pregnancy because of rupture of the amniotic sac. By the second trimester, the risk of miscarriage drops to between 1 in 300 and 1 in 500.[7] When amniocentesis is performed in the later stage of pregnancy, the potential for rupture of the amniotic sac is of less concern because a safe delivery is almost always possible.

Cramping and vaginal bleeding
Some women experience cramping when the needle enters the uterus, and a small amount of vaginal bleeding during or immediately following the amniocentesis. Clients should be instructed to contact their health care provider if the vaginal bleeding or uterine cramping lasts more than several hours.

Needle injury to the fetus
During the amniocentesis, the fetus may inadvertently move into the path of the needle. Serious needle injuries are extremely rare.

Amniotic fluid leak
Rarely, amniotic fluid may leak through the vagina following amniocentesis. For most women, the leak seals and pregnancy proceeds normally.

Rh sensitization
Rarely does an amniocentesis result in fetal blood cells entering the woman's circulation. If the client is Rh negative, she is given Rh immunoglobulin after the amniocentesis to prevent antibody production against her baby's blood.

Infection

Only rarely does an amniocentesis result in a uterine infection. Any client who undergoes an amniocentesis should be instructed to notify her health care provider if she develops a fever.

The Amniocentesis Procedure

There are no food or fluid restrictions before amniocentesis. The woman's bladder must be full before the procedure, so encourage her to increase her fluid intake and not urinate before the procedure. An ultrasound is used to determine the fetus's exact location in the uterus. The use of ultrasound reduces the risk of accidentally puncturing the client's bladder, or the fetus. Typically, an anesthetic is not used for amniocentesis. Inform the client that she may feel some mild discomfort during the procedure, similar to having blood drawn. Guided by ultrasound, the health care provider inserts a thin, hollow needle through the abdominal wall into the uterus. A small amount of amniotic fluid (about an ounce) is withdrawn into a syringe, and the needle removed. The entire procedure usually takes about an hour, but most of that time is because of the ultrasound examination. Reassure the client that her body naturally replaces the small amount of amniotic fluid that has been removed, usually within 3 to 4 hours following the procedure.

After the Amniocentesis Procedure

Ultrasound may be used to monitor the fetal heart rate for a short period after the procedure. Suggest a period of rest after the procedure. Most women are able to resume their normal activities later the same or the following day.

ARTHROCENTESIS

Arthrocentesis, also referred to as a "joint or joint fluid aspiration," "joint tap," or "synovial fluid aspiration,"[8] involves using a needle and syringe to drain or sample synovial fluid from a joint. It is most commonly performed as an office procedure or at the client's bedside, and is used to help determine the cause of joint swelling or arthritis. There are a number of common sites for arthrocentesis including the knee, shoulder, ankle, wrist, elbow, hip, metacarpal and metatarsal phalanges, and temporomandibular joint.

Risks Associated with Arthrocentesis Procedures

Risks and complications related to arthrocentesis are very rare, but may include bruising at the puncture site, bleeding into the joint, and infection. Instruct the client to report any fever, increase in pain, redness, warmth, swelling, and sensation of pressure or drainage from the puncture site.

Arthrocentesis Procedure and Aftercare

When assisting with an arthrocentesis procedure, that are some important considerations to keep in mind. The client should be positioned for optimal visualization according to the joint being aspirated, while taking into consideration the client's physical comfort, privacy, and safety. After anesthetizing the site, the health care provider uses a needle and syringe to access the joint and withdraw any fluid. On occasion during an arthrocentesis, anti-inflammatory medications, such as cortisone, may be injected into the joint to relieve symptoms of inflammation. Once the synovial fluid has been removed, direct pressure is applied to the site for approximately 5 minutes, and a dressing or bandage placed over the puncture site. An ace bandage may be indicated for additional support, and resting or restricting movement of the joint for the next 24 hours is recommended. Inform the client that ice may be applied over the joint for 20 to 30 minutes every 3 to 4 hours for pain or discomfort and, unless contraindicated, the client may also take aspirin, acetaminophen, or other medications as directed or prescribed by their health care provider.

LUMBAR PUNCTURE

Commonly called a lumbar puncture, spinal tap, or spinal puncture, centesis of cerebrospinal fluid (CSF) located within the subarachnoid space of the spinal canal is performed for a number of reasons, including confirming a diagnosis of subarachnoid hemorrhage, metastatic brain cancer, or such infections as meningitis and Lyme disease.[9] Lumbar punctures are also an adjunct in the diagnosis of multiple sclerosis and Guillain-Barré syndrome.[10] In some cases, a lumbar puncture provides access for the introduction of therapeutic agents including antibiotics, chemotherapy, anesthetics, and contrast agents. Lumbar punctures may be performed at the bedside, in the critical care unit, or in the emergency department. Contraindications to lumbar puncture include infection of the skin at the puncture site and increased intracranial pressure. A lumbar puncture should never be performed on a client with increased intracranial pressure because this can result in brain herniation.

Positioning for a lumbar puncture is important for access to the lumbar vertebrae. This procedure may be done either with the client lying down or sitting up. In the lateral recumbent position (**Fig. 1**), instruct the client to lie on either side with the knees flexed toward the chest and the head tucked toward the knees. Explain that this "fetal position" increases the space between the vertebrae and eases insertion of the needle. Placing a pillow under the head may help alleviate any discomfort because this keeps the head on the same plane as the vertebral axis. The client may need assistance to remain in this position until the procedure is completed. If the client is sitting up, have the client lean forward over the bedside table with the head and chest bent toward the knees, and the arms folded over the head. A pillow may be used to cushion the head.

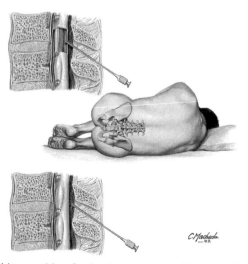

Fig. 1. Lateral decubitus position for lumbar puncture. (*Reprinted from* Netter Anatomy Illustration Collection, © Elsevier Inc. All Rights Reserved.)

For many clients, the thought of having a needle inserted into their spine is terrifying. Clients may experience anxiety more than pain when undergoing a lumbar puncture, especially if they also are anticipating hearing devastating news. In these cases, administering a sedative may be appropriate before beginning the procedure. Inform the client that the entire procedure typically takes about 45 minutes, and that once completed, the client needs to lie flat for an additional period of time.

The Lumbar Puncture Procedure

After the local anesthetic is injected, the health care provider introduces a spinal needle with stylet into the intervertebral space, below the level where the spinal cord terminates, between the 3rd and 4th or 4th and 5th lumbar vertebrae. A small amount of CSF, which normally is clear and colorless, begins to drip from the needle following removal of the stylet. The health care provider measures the client's CSF pressure initially, and at intervals, using a manometer and three-way stopcock. CSF samples are collected, typically in three separate tubes. The tubes should be numbered in the order of collection. The presence of blood in the first tube and no others is likely the result of trauma from the puncture. Blood in all three tubes is a positive sign for subarachnoid hemorrhage. Following removal of the needle, the puncture site should be covered with a small occlusive adhesive bandage.

Following the Lumbar Puncture Procedure

In addition to assessing the client before and during the procedure, the critical care nurse continues to monitor the client thoroughly after the procedure. Along with vital signs and cardiovascular and respiratory status, the assessment should include the client's lower extremity motor and sensory function or any difficulty voiding. Changes in sensory or motor function or voiding following lumbar puncture may indicate transient spinal nerve irritation. If these changes are persistent, this may indicate nerve damage or development of a spinal hematoma. Postprocedure, the client needs to remain in a supine position for 1 to 4 hours. This position prevents leakage of CSF from the puncture site. About 40% of clients develop a frontal headache following lumbar puncture as a result of CSF leaking from the internal puncture site.[11] There is no compelling evidence that prolonged bed rest (up to 12 hours) prevents or reduces the incidence of headache postlumbar puncture.[12,13] Fluids, either oral or intravenous, minimize the risk of dehydration and may help lessen the discomfort associated with the headache, as can the use of mild analgesics. Fluids are thought to help the body replenish its CSF, although research supporting or refuting this practice is lacking.[14]

PARACENTESIS

Paracentesis, also known as "abdominocentesis," "celiocentesis," or "abdominal tap," is a procedure in which excess fluid in the peritoneal space of the abdomen is aspirated through a needle. The fluid is called ascites, abdominal fluid, or peritoneal fluid. Paracentsis can be done in an outpatient setting, the emergency department, or critical care unit. It is typically performed to examine the ascitic fluid and determine the cause of newly diagnosed ascites, or monitor the condition of clients with known ascites. Therapeutically, paracentesis is done to provide relief to the client from the pressure of the excessive fluid in the abdominal cavity. Paracentesis can be helpful in the detection of a perforated viscus in a client with an acute-abdomen, or as a component of differential diagnosis following blunt trauma to the abdomen. Abdominal ultrasound can often detect the presence of fluid in the peritoneal cavity, and during a physical examination percussion over the abdomen results in a dull sound.

The most common causes of ascites include liver disease (primarily cirrhosis) and malignant abdominal masses; however, nephrotic syndrome and heart failure are also associated with the formation of ascites.[15] Ascites results from several different mechanisms. For example, when blood albumin levels are low, osmotic pressure changes allow fluid to shift from blood vessels into the abdominal cavity. In the presence of portal hypertension, high pressure in the portal vein results in increased venous congestion and fluid leakage into the abdominal cavity. Regardless of the cause, clients with ascites usually have a poor prognosis for long-term survival, with 5-year survival rates between 30% and 40%.[16]

The client likely exhibits symptoms before the paracentesis, which may vary depending on the amount of abdominal fluid, and the etiology of the ascites. Most clients have some abdominal distention, and in some the abdomen may be so filled with fluid that the abdominal wall is stretched tight. The client may also be experiencing shortness of breath, a feeling of fullness, decreased appetite, and swollen ankles. Pain is not usually present when the ascites is caused by cirrhosis, but may be present if a malignancy is the causative factor.[17] In addition to vital signs, before this procedure the client must be weighed and the abdominal girth should be measured and recorded. Many agencies encourage "marking" the area where the measurement is taken to maintain consistency.

Conditions that may prohibit paracentesis, or increase the relative risk to the client, include intestinal obstruction; pregnancy, because of the risk of puncturing the uterus; pneumoperitoneum, in which case surgery might be indicated; and infection of the abdominal wall. Additionally, a client who is unlikely or unable to be cooperative, or who has a history of multiple abdominal surgeries, is not a good candidate for this procedure.

The Risks Associated with Paracentesis

Some of the risks associated with the procedure include inadvertent puncture of the intestine or bladder, hypotension related to fluid shifts, leaking of fluid from the puncture site, and rarely intra-abdominal bleeding and infection. The risk of serious bleeding or puncturing the intestine or bladder is low, less than 3%. Have the client void before the procedure because this decreases the chance of bladder puncture. If there were any preprocedural laboratories, such as hematocrit, platelet count, or prothrombin time, make sure they are obtained within 24 to 48 hours before the paracentesis. These are helpful in identifying clients at risk for bleeding complications, and in providing a baseline for comparison should bleeding or blood loss occur after the procedure.

The Paracentesis Procedure

The client may be positioned in bed with the head elevated 45 to 90 degrees, or the client may be required to lay in a slightly recumbent position and turned slightly toward the side selected for the paracentesis. Both of these positions facilitate fluid accumulation in the lower abdomen. Occasionally, the client might have to change positions to further facilitate drainage of the fluid. A site is selected beneath the umbilicus, and is prepared with an antiseptic solution. An anesthetic is injected. Explain that as the paracentesis needle is inserted into the abdomen, there may be a temporary feeling of sharp pain or pressure. Also explain that fluid samples may be collected and sent for laboratory analysis. Typically, these tests include cell counts, cytology, and cultures. Depending on the purpose of the paracentesis, the health care provider withdraws as much fluid as necessary and safely possible. Large-volume abdominal paracentesis with removal of 4 to 6 L of fluid is considered safe and more than 5 L of fluid is standard therapy.[18] Removal of greater than 10 L should be performed no more often than every 2 weeks.[19] If it is anticipated that a large amount of fluid will be removed, a tubing and stopcock may be attached to regulate the flow of fluid.

Withdrawing the fluid slowly avoids fluid shifts and may minimize any drop in blood pressure. Anticipate that the client may require IV fluids or a colloid, such as albumin, to prevent or treat hypotension or shock. When the fluid has been drained, the needle is removed and the puncture site covered with a small gauze dressing and bandage. Typically, paracentesis takes about 20 to 30 minutes. In cases where a large amount of fluid is removed, the procedure may take longer.

Following the Paracentesis Procedure

After the procedure, observe the client for continued leakage of fluid or bleeding. The client should lie supine such that the puncture site is "elevated" for at least an hour to allow the puncture site to close. Explain that they may continue to have some clear fluid drain from the puncture site, especially if a large amount was removed. The drainage should diminish, however, within 1 to 2 days.

Nursing responsibilities after the procedure include monitoring for hypovolemia and electrolyte abnormalities.[20] In some clients, the blood pressure may drop during or immediately after the procedure, and remain low for several days following the procedure. In these cases, clients need to be instructed not to stand up or move about too quickly. In some extreme cases, the blood pressure may also need to be monitored at home. The client should be instructed to report a fever, increasing abdominal pain, dizziness, or feelings of being light-headed. They should also report any blood in their urine, redness around the puncture site, or any fluid leak that persists for greater than 2 days. The nurse should weigh, and the abdominal girth remeasured, following the same procedure and location as the preprocedure measurement. Vital signs should be measured periodically for about an hour postprocedure. Unless otherwise directed, clients may resume their normal activities as tolerated following the procedure.

PERICARDIOCENTESIS

To understand the dynamics of a pericardiocentesis, it is helpful to think of the pericardium as a two-layered sac that encloses the heart. The inner layer is called the visceral pericardium; the outer (and tougher) layer is called the parietal pericardium. Normally, the pericardial sac contains about 20 to 30 mL of fluid, which cushions and lubricates the heart during systole. The client may have a medical condition, such as an infection, heart failure, or cancer, which can cause an increase in the amount of pericardial fluid. Abnormal amounts of fluid may also be the result of pericarditis, trauma, surgery, invasive heart procedures, myocardial infarction, and renal failure. When excessive fluid accumulates in the pericardial sac, it is referred to as a pericardial "effusion." Signs and symptoms of pericardial effusion include anxiety and restlessness, tachycardia, difficulty breathing and tachypnea, a pericardial friction rub, and chest pain. Pericardiocentesis, also referred to as a "pericardial tap," involves removing the excess fluid from the pericardial sac, and is instrumental in determining the etiology of the effusion and in alleviating any symptoms associated with the effusion.

Cardiac Tamponade

A pericardioentesis may also be performed on an emergency basis to treat cardiac tamponade. Cardiac tamponade is a rare and life-threatening condition that occurs from a rapid or excessive accumulation of fluid (usually blood) in the pericardial sac. The excess fluid impedes the ability of the heart to fill properly and prevents the ventricles from pumping effectively (**Fig. 2**). Because cardiac tamponade is a potentially fatal condition, pericardiocentesis can be a life-saving procedure.

Cardiac tamponade can occur following chest trauma, open heart surgery, or a penetrating chest injury. Acute cardiac tamponade is one of the most serious complications of catheter-based interventional procedures, and has been reported as both an early and late complication of pacemaker implantation with the use of fixation leads.[21–23] In addition to the symptoms associated with a pericardial effusion, patients experiencing cardiac tamponade likely are hypotensive and have muffled heart sounds and jugular venous distention (Beck triad). If experiencing cardiac tamponade, the client needs IV fluids to increase the preload of the heart, which increases ventricular filling. In many cases, vasopressors, such as dopamine hydrocloride may also be required.

Risks Associated with Pericardiocentesis

As with any invasive procedure, there are risks associated with pericardiocentesis. With the use of guided imaging techniques, however, the incidence of complications has improved. Echocardiography, for example, assists the health care provider as they guide the needle and catheter into the pericardial sac, and avoid trauma to the heart and coronary arteries. Currently, about 5% of patients undergoing pericardiocentesis experience a major complication.[24] Possible complications include puncture of the myocardium or coronary artery; myocardial infarction; cardiac arrhythmias; pneumopericardium; infection (pericarditis); and accidental puncture of the stomach, lung, or liver.

The Pericardiocentesis Procedure

Pericardiocentesis may be performed as an outpatient procedure, in the emergency department, at the bedside in the ICU, or in the cardiac catheterization suite. The client does not need be NPO for a pericardiocentesis; however, if undergoing an elective diagnostic or therapeutic pericardiocentesis, the client should restrict food and oral

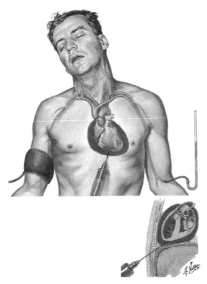

Fig. 2. Pericardial tamponade. (*Reprinted from* Netter Anatomy Illustration Collection, © Elsevier Inc. All Rights Reserved.)

fluids for several[2-6] hours before the procedure. An echocardiogram is done to identify the size and location of the effusion. An IV line, if not already placed, needs to be started for administration of any fluids or medications that may need to be given. The critical care nurse should closely monitor the client's vital signs, especially blood pressure and electrocardiogram. Continuous cardiac monitoring allows the nurse to continually assess the client's heart rate and rhythm, and observe for development of any arrhythmias. Oxygen should also be applied, and as a precautionary measure, defibrillator pads may be applied. The client and the client's family should be informed that the procedure normally takes between 20 and 60 minutes.

The client should be positioned in semi-Fowler position with the head of the bed raised 30 to 60 degrees. Placement in semi-Fowler position lowers the diaphragm and other abdominal organs, and facilitates the fluid pooling at the apex of the heart. Unless the procedure is being performed emergently, the client is mildly sedated and a local anesthetic injected over the area of the chest where the needle is inserted, typically at the junction of the xiphoid process and left costal arch. The health care provider uses a 5- to 6-in long cardiac needle, inserts it at a 30- to 45-degree angle just below the xiphoid, and advances it toward the client's left shoulder while gently aspirating on the syringe. Explain to the client that he or she may experience some pressure as the needle enters the pericardial sac. When the sac is penetrated, there is a flashback of fluid or blood noted in the needle hub. Normal pericardial fluid should be clear and colorless to straw colored. If the pericardiocentesis is being performed for diagnostic purposes, several samples of the pericardial fluid are collected and sent for analysis. If there is a significant amount of fluid that needs to be removed, or if there are indications that the fluid will reaccumulate, a pericardial catheter may be attached to the needle to allow for continuous drainage into a collection bag.

For some clients who experience episodes of fluid reaccumulation requiring repeat pericardiocentesis procedures, such medications as tetracycline and bleomycin can be injected into the pericardial sac. This process is known as "pericardiodesis." These medications act as irritants or sclerosing agents, which cause the pericardium to scar and adhere to the surface of the heart, preventing any further accumulation of fluid in the pericardial space.

After the Pericardiocentesis

After the needle is withdrawn, pressure must be applied to the insertion site for approximately 5 minutes to control any bleeding. A small dressing or bandage is then used to cover and protect the site. Typically, postprocedural assessment includes continual electrocardiogram monitoring for changes or premature ventricular contractions, vital sign measurement, assessing for jugular vein distention, and observing the puncture site for any bleeding. Some clients, if not already in the ICU, may be admitted there for observation following a pericardiocentesis. At the time of discharge, instruct the client to inspect the site for bleeding or signs of infection (redness, swelling, drainage) until the site has healed.

THORACENTESIS

Similar to the heart, each lung is also enclosed in two membranes. The visceral pleura adheres to the surface of the lung, and the parietal pleura lines the inner surface of the chest wall. The area between these membranes is called the "pleural space" or "cavity." A small amount of serous fluid normally fills this space, which serves to decrease friction between the lung and chest wall during respiration. When an excessive amount of pleural fluid accumulates in the space, it is called a "pleural effusion."

Imaging techniques, such as chest radiograph, CT, or ultrasound, in addition to the physical examination findings (maximum site of dullness to percussion), are used to confirm the location of the pleural effusion. The client may have a condition, such as a lung infection or tumor, heart failure, cancer, or kidney disease, all of which can cause a pleural effusion. A thoracentesis, also known as a "pleural tap" or "pleural fluid aspiration," is performed to obtain a sample of pleural fluid for analysis and diagnosis. A thoracentesis is also used therapeutically to drain a pleural effusion or instill medication. Any condition that results in a large amount of pleural fluid accumulating in the pleural space usually requires removal to facilitate breathing. Some clients may only need a thoracentesis as a one-time event while the underlying condition is being treated. For malignant pleural effusions, however, especially if the patient is frail or with poor life expectancy, thoracentesis may need to be done more frequently.[25]

Thoracentesis can be safely performed at the patient's bedside, as an outpatient procedure, in an emergency department, or in a critical care unit. The procedure typically takes about 30 minutes. Instruct the client that no special preparation or food or fluid restrictions are required. There are no absolute contraindications to thoracentesis, other than the client's refusal or inability to consent to the procedure. There are special considerations for clients who have any uncontrolled coughing, coagulopathy, or anatomic alterations of the chest. These conditions are associated with increase risks during the procedure.

Risks Associated with Thoracentesis

Complications from thoracentesis are uncommon, but some risks are involved. They include pneumothorax, pain, bleeding, bruising, or infection at the needle insertion site; pulmonary edema; reaccumulation of fluid; and very rarely, accidental puncture of the liver or spleen because of an unusually deep needle insertion. The indications for a thoracentesis clearly slant the benefit/risk ratio in favor of the benefits of this procedure.

The Thoracentesis Procedure

During the procedure it is important for the client to try to avoid coughing, to avoid breathing deeply, and to remain still during the procedure. The client should understand that any excessive movement increases the risk of needle contact with the lung or can result in needle dislodgment. The client should be encouraged actually to hum out loud because this prevents deep breathing, which expands the lung, and it decreases the risk of needle contact with the lung. Obtain baseline vital signs including a pulse oximetry reading. Continually assess for signs and symptoms of respiratory distress during the procedure. If a large pleural effusion is present, the client likely is experiencing difficulty breathing. Auscultate and document the quality and type of breath sounds especially noting adventitious, absent, or decreased sounds on the affected side.

The selection of a site for thoracentesis has traditionally been guided by chest radiograph and physical examination findings. Recent evidence indicates, however, that chest ultrasound guidance improves both site selection and needle insertion, so much so that some experts are now recommending its routine use for thoracentesis.[25-27] In addition, although available in most institutions, direct monitoring of pleural pressure during therapeutic thoracentesis is not widely used because most thoracentesis procedures are performed at the bedside.[28]

Assist the client to be seated upright on the side of the bed with the head and folded arms resting on a pillow on the overbed table. A recumbent or supine thoracentesis can be performed on patients who are ventilated or unable to tolerate sitting up by turning and positioning them on the unaffected side, and with the arm of the affected side raised above the head. The head of the bed should still be elevated 30 to 40 degrees. These positions expand the intercostal space for the needle insertion.[29] Once the skin is anesthetized, a larger needle and syringe containing additional anesthetic are inserted at the upper border of the rib that is one intercostal space below the fluid level at the midscapular line. While periodically aspirating, the health care provider advances the needle and injects the anesthetic at progressively deeper levels. Once the needle has penetrated the parietal pleura (the most painful part), and pleural fluid is able to be aspirated, the depth of the needle is noted. A thoracentesis needle-catheter with three-way stopcock and 30- to 50-mL syringe attached is then inserted to the depth noted during introduction of the anesthetic. Typically, the needle is removed to reduce the risk of pneumothorax. Any pleural fluid may then be aspirated with the syringe, or tubing can be connected to the catheter, which allows the fluid to flow by gravity into a collection bottle or bag (**Fig. 3**). The amount of fluid removed depends on the client's clinical scenario. The fluid is removed slowly and no more than 1.5 L in any 24-hour period is drained. This minimizes the risk of developing re-expansion pulmonary edema and hypotension. It is theorized, although the exact mechanism is unknown, that as the lung rapidly reinflates, it creates a reperfusion injury to the alveolar capillaries, increasing their permeability and leading to pulmonary edema and hypoxia. An important nursing consideration regarding this potential complication is that some clients may require intubation and mechanical ventilation.

Explain to the client that in cases where the client experiences severe pain, develops bradycardia, or has increased difficulty breathing, the procedure may be halted. These symptoms may indicate development of complications, such as hypovolemic shock, tension pneumothorax, or cardiac distress. Inform the client that it is also possible that no fluid is removed during the thoracentesis. This is referred to as a "dry tap" and may be caused by using a needle that is too short, inserting it too high, or when no fluid was actually present in the pleural space.[30]

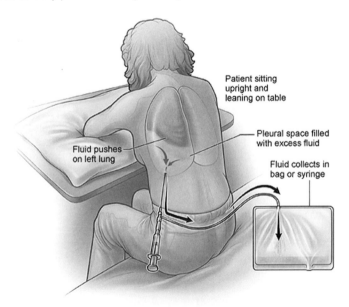

Fig. 3. Thoracentesis. (*From* National Heart, Lung and Blood Institute. Diseases and conditions index. Available at http://www.nhlbi.nih.gov/health/dci/Diseases/thor/thor_whatis.html.)

A thoracentesis may also be done before another procedure called "pleurodesis." During this procedure, a chemical or medication sclerosing agent (ie, talc or doxycycline) is instilled into the pleural space. This triggers an inflammatory reaction over the surface of the lung and inside the pleural space, which causes the visceral and parietal pleurae to adhere together. This eliminates the space between the two pleural membranes and prevents or reduces the collection of additional pleural fluid. Pleurodesis may be recommended for a client whose pleural effusion has occurred more than one time.

After the Thoracentesis

A pressure dressing should be applied over the puncture site after the catheter is withdrawn. Assess the site for any drainage and monitor the client's vital signs per institutional protocol. Current evidence suggests that repeating the chest radiograph postthoracentesis is not indicated, unless the patient is symptomatic.[27] Observe for signs and symptoms of respiratory distress, and assess for the development of additional symptoms including chest discomfort or pain and cough. As the client's lung reexpands following fluid removal, a cough may develop. The client may experience some hemoptysis following the procedure. Provide reassurance that this is normal, but that the primary health care provider should be notified for any increasing shortness of breath or chest pain. The client may also complain of pain with respiration, especially if the process that led to development of the effusion involved an inflammatory process. This pleuritic pain is a result of the parietal and visceral pleurae approximating following the fluid removal. Note that a pleural friction rub may be heard when auscultating the client's lung sounds. Most clients having an outpatient thoracentesis can usually return home after a 30- to 60-minute period of observation postprocedure.

SUMMARY

Nursing actions and considerations before and during selected centesis procedures, and components of appropriate aftercare, are foundational to caring for clients undergoing any centesis procedures. As a critical care nurse, knowledge about why and how centesis studies are performed, and the role and responsibility in assisting with these procedures, increases the client's safety and contributes to improving the overall outcome.

REFERENCES

1. The free dictionary. Available at: http://www.thefreedictionary.com/centesis. Accessed February 22, 2009.
2. Available at: http://www.wordinfo.info/words/index/info. Accessed February 22, 2009.
3. American College of Obstetricians and Gynecologists (ACOG). Invasive prenatal testing for aneuploidy. ACOG Practice Bulletin Dec 2007;88. Available at: http://www.guideline.gov/summary/summary.aspx?ss=15&doc_id=12629&nbr=6537&string=#s23.
4. Available at: http://www.marchofdimes.com/professionals/14332_1164.asp. Accessed May 15, 2009.
5. Available at: http://www.mayoclinic.com/health/amniocentesis/MY00155/DSECTION=results. Accessed May 15, 2009.
6. Luo G, Norwitz ER. Revisiting amniocentesis for fetal lung maturity after 36 weeks' gestation. Rev Obstet Gynecol 2008;1(2):61–8.
7. Available at: http://video.about.com/pregnancy/Amniocentesis.htm. Accessed May 15, 2009.

8. Arthrocentesis-joint fluid aspiration. Available at: http://www.steadyhealth.com/srticles/Arthrocentesis_Joint_fluid-aspiration-a417-f33.h. Accessed February 22, 2009.
9. Sucholeiki R, Waldman AL. Lumbar puncture (CSF examination) 2006. Available at: http://www.emedicine.com/neuro/topic557htm. Accessed March 2, 2009.
10. Barker E. Neuroscience nursing: a spectrum of care. 2nd edition. St. Louis (MO): Mosby; 2002.
11. Rushing J. LP clinical do's & don'ts: assisting with lumbar puncture. Nursing 2007;37(1):23.
12. Ahmed SV, Jayawarna C, Jude E. Post lumber puncture headache: diagnosis and management. Postgrad Med J 2006;82(973):713–6.
13. McLafferty FA. Lumbar puncture. Nurs Stand 2008;22:46–8.
14. Ignatavicius D, Workman ML, editors. Medical surgical nursing. 5th edition. St. Louis (MO): Elsevier Saunders; 2006. p. 942.
15. Glickman RM. Abdominal swelling and ascites. In: Fauci AS, editor. Harrison's principles of internal medicine. New York: McGraw-Hill; 1998. p. 256–7.
16. Ginès P, Cárdenos A, Arroyo V, et al. Management of cirrhosis and ascites. N Engl J Med 2004;350(16):1646–54.
17. Shah R, Fields J. Ascites 2007. Available at: http://www.emedicine.com/med/topiclZS.htm. Accessed March 2, 2009.
18. Sargent S. Hepatology: the management and nursing care of cirrhotic ascites. Br J Nurs 2006;15:212–9.
19. Yeung E, Wong FS. The management of cirrhotic ascites. MedGenMed 2002;4(4):8.
20. Heitkemper MM, Croghan A, Cox-North P. Liver, pancreas and biliary problems. In: Lewis SL, Heitkemper MM, Dirksen SR, et al, editors. Medical-surgical nursing: assessment and management of clinical problems. 7th edition. St. Louis (MO): Mosby; 2007. p. 1110–4.
21. Aizawa K, Kaneko Y, Yamagishi T, et al. Oozing from the pericardium as an etiology of cardiac tamponade associated with screw-in atrial leads. Pacing Clin Electrophysiol 2001;24:381–3.
22. Velavan P, Chauhan A. An unusual presentation of delayed cardiac perforation caused by atrial screw-in lead. Heart 2003;89:364.
23. Ellenbogen KA, Wood MA, Shepard RK. Delayed complications following pacemaker implantation. Pacing Clin Electrophysiol 2002;25:1155–8.
24. WebMD Pericardiocentesis. Reference provided in collaboration with the Cleveland Clinic. Available at: http://www.webmd.com/heart-disease/guide/pericardiocentesis. Accessed February 22, 2009.
25. Heffner JE, Klein JS. Recent advances in the diagnosis and management of malignant pleural effusions. Mayo Clin Proc 2008;83(2):235–50.
26. Buchanan DR, Neville E. Thoracoscopy for physicians: a practical guide. London: Hodder Arnold; 2004.
27. The Merck manual of patient symptoms. Thoracentesis: diagnostic and therapeutic pulmonary procedures. Available at: http://www.merck.com/mmpe/sec05/ch047/ch047i.html. Accessed February 22, 2009.
28. Feller-Kopman D, Walkey A, Berkowitz D, et al. The relationship of pleural pressure to symptom development during therapeutic thoracentesis. Chest 2006;129:1556–60.
29. Perry AG, Potter PA, editors. Clinical nursing skills and techniques. 7th edition. St. Louis (MO): Mosby; 2010. p. 1176–82.
30. Light RW. Pleural diseases. 5th edition. Philadelphia: Lippincott Williams & Wilkins; 2007.

Urodynamics

Tamara M. Robertson, MSN, APN, FNP-BC, CUNP*,
Amy S. Hamlin, MSN, RN

KEYWORDS

• Urodynamics • Stress incontinence • Neurogenic bladder
• Overactive bladder • Voiding dysfunction

A properly functioning urinary system is essential to the body's physical well-being and to a person's general sense of contentment. Urinary dysfunction can be the precipitating cause of pathophysiologic illnesses and psychosocial difficulties in regards to self-esteem and social isolation. Many patients become confined to their homes because of fears of having an embarrassing episode or urinary incontinence.[1] A thorough history and physical of all aspects of patients' physical and mental status should be assessed by the professional nurse, regardless of the setting. If assessment findings uncover a problem with urinary elimination the nurse should make the appropriate referrals with the understanding that urinary elimination alterations may have serious consequences.

OVERVIEW AND HISTORY OF URODYNAMICS

Simply stated, the function of the bladder is twofold: storage and expulsion of urine. Urodynamic studies assess to what extent the bladder and urethra are performing the synchronous function of storing and releasing urine. Unlike other systems that might be evaluated through one very specific diagnostic test or scan, the lower urinary system and its underlying pathologic disorders need to be reproduced to be understood.[2] For a provider to make an accurate diagnosis, specific measurements and observations of lower urinary function must be made. Through interaction between the provider and patients, an attempt is made to recreate the clinical symptoms in a laboratory setting. The findings of urodynamic studies assist the provider in uncovering the underlying pathophysiology of the urological problem.[3]

Urodynamic studies have evolved since 1927 when D.K. Rose first introduced the cystometrograph, an instrument designed to determine filling and voiding bladder pressures.[3] Since that time the procedure and the equipment to perform the test have become commercialized and mass produced. However, the basis for the idea of measuring bladder pressures remains much the same as when it was first developed.[3]

School of Nursing, Austin Peay State University, McCord Building 313, PO Box 4658, Clarksville, TN 37044, USA
* Corresponding author.
E-mail address: robertsonm@apsu.edu (T.M. Robertson).

Crit Care Nurs Clin N Am 22 (2010) 109–120
doi:10.1016/j.ccell.2009.10.001
0899-5885/10/$ – see front matter © 2010 Elsevier Inc. All rights reserved.

Urodynamics may be helpful in determining the specific cause of patients' lower urinary tract symptoms. In addition to patients' history, physical, voiding diary, and pad count, this test is used to assist in determining the causes of incontinence, urinary frequency, hesitancy and urgency, a sense of incomplete emptying, urinary retention, and various other urologic complaints.

The procedure is performed either at the bedside, or in an outpatient setting, usually without anesthesia. There are also ambulatory urodynamics in which patients may have a portable option under more physiologic conditions for longer periods.[4] The provider performing the test is either a physician or a nurse who is educated as an experienced urodynamicist. The idea is to mimic and reproduce the symptoms of the patients' presenting complaint. Therefore, it is important to have the patients' report of sensations and events during the test. Patient education should be performed and an informed consent obtained before the examination. Patients need to have an understanding of the components of the test including the need for urethral catheterization. Patients must present for testing with a full bladder. Prior to testing, patients are advised to omit the use of lotions, powder, or sprays to the pelvic area. Various types of equipment are used in the testing and specific equipment varies based upon individual manufacturers (**Fig. 1**). No matter which manufacturer produces the equipment, all have the same resultant outcomes. The difference is found only in the instruments of measurement and computer programming (see **Fig. 1**).

Because of the invasive nature of testing, a potential post-procedure complication is the development of a urinary tract infection (UTI). A urinalysis to assess for bacteriuria should be obtained on all patients before urodynamic testing. Risks to patients with an active UTI undergoing urodynamics include potential introduction of infection from the lower urinary tract to the upper urinary tract.[5] Studies have shown prophylactic

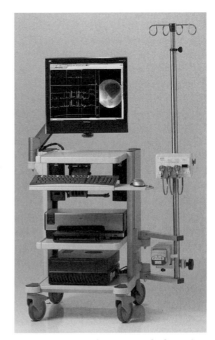

Fig. 1. Example of urodynamic equipment. (*Courtesy of* Life-Tech International, Stafford, TX.)

antibiotics reduce the risk for post-procedure bacteriuria[6]; however, there is no standard of practice for all providers. Therefore, the use of prophylactic antibiotic use before urodynamics is usually based on practitioner preference, though most clinicians routinely prescribe prophylactic antibiotics for high-risk groups.[6]

NORMAL MICTURITION

Before going into detail regarding urodynamics, the discussion and understanding of the normal process of micturition, the act of voiding, should be obtained. The bladder is a hollow vessel used in the filling, storage, and emptying of the waste product urine. The bladder is capable of accomplishing storage of urine without pain or conscious effort.[7] Once full continence is achieved, normally during the toddler or preschool period, the following micturition process occurs. The storage of urine is accomplished by the sympathetic nervous system as it sends messages to the bladder that cause the detrusor muscle, the primary muscle in the bladder, to relax and the internal sphincter to constrict.[1] This process allows for urine filling/storage. As the bladder expands, stretch receptors are stimulated and the person feels the urge to void. In a normal adult this occurs at approximately 200 to 300 mL.[1] Though the urge to void may occur at 200 to 300 mL, the average maximum bladder capacity is 400 to 550 mL.[8] Once the bladder fills, the parasympathetic nervous system sends impulses that cause the detrusor muscle to contract and the internal sphincter to relax, which results in the emptying of the bladder. This process is extremely important not only to the lower urinary tract but also to the upper urinary tract. Urinary bladder abnormalities that affect bladder compliance, the ability of the bladder to expand and maintain low intravesical pressures, may negatively affect the upper urinary tract ultimately resulting in renal failure.

COMPONENTS OF URODYNAMICS

Urodynamics consists of multiple steps to put the pieces together to discover a complete clinical picture. Each step adds more information in assisting and determining the diagnosis, and ultimately a reasonable treatment plan for patients. Much like critical care nurses who use electrocardiography to monitor the electrical conduction of the cardiac muscle, the urologist or urologic nurse can use multichannel urodynamics to determine the function of the bladder.

Uroflowmetry

Uroflowmetry tests the volume of urine released, the speed at which it is excreted, and the length of the excretion. Uroflowmetry provides an objective assessment of voiding dysfunction. Through voiding in a special toilet attached to a monitored collection device, the provider can determine how many ml/s on average patients void. In addition, uroflowmetry also records the highest rate obtained during a particular void (Qmax) and the time to Qmax.[9] Obstruction is likely if Qmax is less than 10 mL per second.[10] Limitations of this test involve a low sensitivity, yet a high specificity.[9] Also, the test must be considered and interpreted with caution if patients void less than 100 to 150 mL.[3]

Post-void Residual

After patients void during uroflowmetry, the provider must determine if any residual urine remains in the bladder. Determining the post-void residual (PVR) after the completion of the uroflowmetry is the next step in the evaluation. This is either done with ultrasound or through catheterization. If patients are to undergo the entire battery of tests included in the urodynamic studies, then it is reasonable to obtain PVR through catheterization. Cole and Dmochowski state, "In adults, it is suggested that a value of less than 25 mL is considered normal and one greater than 100 mL warrants careful surveillance or treatment."[3]

Multichannel Filling Cystometry

A cystometrogram measures how much fluid the bladder can hold, how much pressure the bladder can withstand as it fills, and at what level of filling patients feels the urge to void. Cystometry testing is accomplished by insertion of a 10 Fr or less urethral catheter with pressure measuring capabilities on the proximal end of the catheter (**Fig. 2**). If the practitioner is using a double lumen catheter, one lumen is used to measure intravesical pressure (Pves) and the other lumen is used to fill the bladder with 0.9% normal saline or contrast medium if fluoroscopy is being used. The filling medium may either be warmed or at room temperature. Filling should occur at a rate of 10 to 100 mL/min (see **Fig. 2**).

An additional single lumen catheter is placed either in the vagina or rectum. This catheter has a balloon on the proximal end filled with a small amount of H_2O. This catheter has the capability to measure intra-abdominal pressure (Pabd). The difference between Pves (the pressure reading from the catheter in the bladder) and Pabd (the pressure reading from the catheter in the vagina or rectum) determines the detrusor pressure (Pdet). The detrusor pressure of an empty bladder should normally be 0 cm/H_2O. Having knowledge of the detrusor pressure, the practitioner will witness the intravesical pressure and detrusor muscle activity in a graph form. This knowledge provides valuable information to assist in the diagnosis of bladder dysfunction and the formulation of an appropriate treatment plan.

During the filling phase of the assessment, bladder compliance is also evaluated. As discussed previously, as the normal bladder distends, maintenance of steady low pressures throughout filling occurs (Pves <10cm/H_2O).[8] However, in some cases the bladder may be dysfunctional and this low pressure filling does not occur. This dysfunction is detected during filling phase cystometry, as the bladder fills, Pves rises at an unacceptable rate. This is termed poor bladder compliance. If Pves rises to 40 cm/H_2O or more it is associated with upper urinary tract deterioration.[3] As is standard practice with any catheterization, the practitioner must maintain sterile technique throughout this procedure.

Leak Point Pressure

With the Pves and Pabd catheters in place, patients are instructed to increase the intra-abdominal pressure by performing valsalva maneuvers, coughing, or other methods. The urodynamicist observes patients for the first leakage and the corresponding Pabd for which this occurred.[11] Extremely low readings (<40 cm/H_2O) are indicative of severe stress urinary incontinence related to sphincteric weakness.[11]

Pressure Flow Study

The pressure flow study assesses the interaction between the bladder, bladder outlet, pelvic floor, and urethra during voiding.[3] A pressure flow study is obtained at the end of filling when patients report a strong urge to void. Patients are instructed to void with the catheters in place using the monitored toilet used during the uroflowmetry study. During voiding, Pves, Pabd, and Pdet are all measured. This portion of the study is useful in determining bladder outlet obstruction and other voiding dysfunctions.

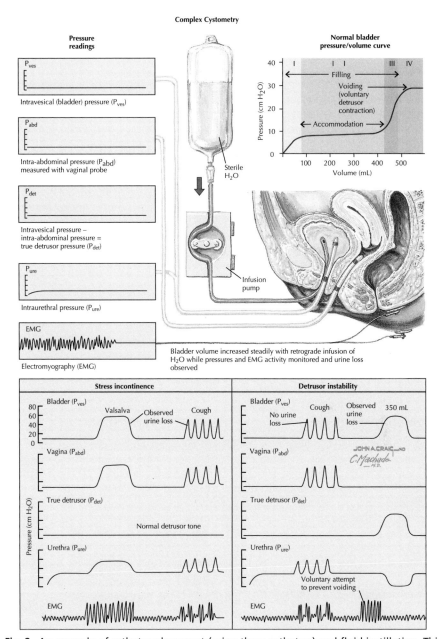

Fig. 2. An example of catheter placement (using three catheters) and fluid instillation. This figure also depicts examples of pressure readings, normal bladder pressure/volume curve, and examples of urodynamic findings in stress incontinence and detrusor instability that occurs with overactive bladder. (*Reprinted from* Netter Atlas of Human Anatomy © Elsevier Inc. All rights reserved.)

Electromyography

Urodynamics may be performed with or without electromyography (EMG). EMG is used to monitor any inappropriate pelvic floor muscle behavior.[12] Specifically, EMG is used to gain information regarding the coordination of the perineal muscles with the detrusor muscle. Electrodes are placed by the anus and may be either needle or self adhesive surface electrodes. EMG is useful in diagnosing urologic problems in patients who have neurologic abnormalities associated with interrupted neural pathways that control micturition. Specific conditions with related problems of urination include spinal cord injury, Parkinson's disease, and multiple sclerosis.

Videourodynamics

Videourodynamics provide a means to perform the urodynamic studies as previously discussed along with visualization of the body structures involved in the lower urinary tract. Many times videourodynamics are not necessary to perform an accurate assessment; however, the simultaneous pressure measurement with fluoroscopy may reduce the possibility of misinterpretation caused by artifact.[13]

POST-PROCEDURE CARE

Following the urodynamic studies, the practitioner must confirm that patients do not have any residual of the instilled medium. If patients have not completely emptied/voided the instilled medium, they must be assessed for residual and PVR obtained through catheterization. Patients should be instructed to report any signs and symptoms of urinary tract infection (UTI). Based upon the urodynamic findings, it is imperative that the patient receive proper follow up with a urology provider.

URINARY INCONTINENCE

Urinary incontinence is a diagnosis that affects men and women of various ages. It is estimated that over 10 million patients suffer with some degree of urinary incontinence and nearly $15 to 20 billion is spent on this diagnosis annually.[11] There are many reasons why a person would be hesitant to discuss this troubling issue with their health care provider. Patients might be embarrassed to discuss their symptoms or they may feel that the symptoms will only be transitory. Elderly patients will commonly accept the incontinence as a normal part of aging and fail to seek help.[11] The term urinary incontinence may be used for many different incontinence symptoms, and depending on the specific underlying pathophysiology, may be transient or become chronic in nature. Despite the mechanism, urinary incontinence is troubling and may have a significant impact on quality of life.

STRESS URINARY INCONTINENCE

Stress urinary incontinence is the complaint of uncontrollable loss of urine with coughing, sneezing, lifting, or straining. The symptoms of stress urinary incontinence vary in significance ranging from occasional drops of urine to more frequent leaking. Stress urinary incontinence is thought to be caused by an increasing intra-abdominal pressure which exceeds the urethral pressure.[14] The leakage is caused by an incompetent continence mechanism at the bladder neck, which is secondary to either urethral hypermobility or intrinsic sphincter deficiency.[8] Female risk factors for stress urinary incontinence include obstetric and gynecologic causes. Women who have a history of multiple pregnancies and deliveries, specifically those complicated by forceps assistance, are at a higher risk for stress urinary incontinence.[15] Other women at risk include those who participate in strenuous exercise or who have increased weight and body mass index (BMI).[14] Postmenopausal women are also at risk because of the occurrence of stress urinary incontinence as the urethra atrophies with a decrease in estrogen production. Men are not immune to stress urinary incontinence. Those with a history of prostate surgery for benign prostatic hyperplasia (BPH) or prostate cancer may also have complaints of stress urinary incontinence.[16]

Diagnosis of stress urinary incontinence is made by a combination of history, physical examination, and laboratory studies. A bladder diary is essential in assisting in the diagnosis of lower urinary tract disorders. The diary is kept over 1 to 7 days during which patients record the amount and type of fluid intake and output and whether they were continent or incontinent.[4] This diary provides additional objective findings to be included in the diagnostic workup. With any lower urinary tract dysfunction, the presence of bacteriuria, pyuria, and hematuria must also be ruled out as an underlying cause of patients' complaints. Urodynamic studies are not used for original diagnosis, but are essential in identifying the specific cause and planning for appropriate treatment.[15] Because patients are not capable of determining whether they suffer from stress urinary incontinence caused by intra-abdominal pressure increases or urge incontinence associated with unstable detrusor contractions, studies of urodynamics are required. Goals and treatment for stress urinary incontinence focus primarily on behavioral interventions including pelvic floor muscle exercises (Kegel's). Other treatment modalities for stress urinary incontinence include biofeedback, use of weighted vaginal devices, electrical stimulation units, and bladder neck support devices.[15] There is little to no pharmacologic intervention for stress urinary incontinence. Postmenopausal women have had positive results with the use of localized intravaginal estrogen.[14] When less invasive treatments are not effective, surgical measures may be used.

Case Report

A 48-year-old postmenopausal woman presents to the clinic with a 2-month history of loss of urine when laughing, sneezing or coughing. She complains that she does not leave home because she is uncomfortable and needs to wear two maxi pads per day, both moderately saturated, to prevent accidents. Voiding diary reveals excessive intake of caffeine and carbonated beverages. Health history includes mild hypertension; BMI of 27; smoking one pack of cigarettes per day for 20 years; and complaints of coughing, especially upon arising. Surgical and obstetric history includes cholecystectomy 3 years ago, vaginal delivery of four children and one cesarean section delivery. Urinalysis is negative for infection. History and physical are otherwise unremarkable.

An urodynamic evaluation is performed to evaluate the mechanism of the incontinence. Findings from the urodynamic study include

- Uroflowmetry: Overall it was within normal limits with a Qmax equal to 25 mL/s.
- Postvoidal residual: PVR equals 25 mL.
- Cystometry: Patient had first desire at 115 mL of filling. Patient had normal desire at 200 mL of filling. Patient had strong desire at 275 mL of filling. Throughout the filling phase, bladder compliance was found to be within normal limits.

- Leak point pressure: At 150 mL of filling, the patient was instructed to perform the valsalva maneuver. Upon straining, the patient had an average valsalva leak point pressure of 48cm/H_2O.
- Pressure flow study: Once patient reported strong desire at 275 mL of filling and she was instructed to void. No abnormalities were identified. Detrusor pressure during voiding was found to be within normal limits.

Based on the urodynamic study, this patient has the diagnosis of stress urinary incontinence. Treatment recommendations for this patient include correct instruction of Kegel's exercises, dietary changes to include decreasing amounts and eventual omission of caffeine intake, and weight loss. The patient will follow up with the urology provider in 3 months to assess outcomes. Should the patient report continuing or worsening symptoms despite progress regarding behavioral compliance, surgical intervention may be considered.

OVERACTIVE BLADDER WITH OR WITHOUT INCONTINENCE

Overactive bladder (OAB) is a symptom-based syndrome characterized by the presence of urinary urgency with or without actual incontinence.[17] Patients experience an extreme desire to void at inappropriate times. Patients who have OAB may also experience frequency of urination, in excess of eight voids per day, and nocturia. Wet and dry OAB can cause a significant reduction in quality of life. One of the most important concerns of health care providers is the morbidity of OAB secondary to falls, fractures, skin infections, and depression.[18] OAB is estimated to affect 33 million citizens globally.[19]

The etiology of OAB is most commonly idiopathic, however, there is a noted relationship with advancing age, cognitive impairment, and neurologic dysfunction.[20] The prevalence in women and men in the United States is 16.9% and 16%, respectively.[19]

A clinical diagnosis may be obtained through a thorough history and physical examination. Patients will likely complain of sudden, frequent urges to void with or without incontinence. Patients should be questioned regarding any triggers of these sudden urges. A urinary diary should be maintained to help in determining a diagnosis of OAB. Female patients must also undergo a physical examination that must include a vaginal examination to confirm or rule out pelvic organ prolapse. An abdominal examination should be performed to assess for any abdominal masses or tenderness. Urodynamics may be used to obtain a more objective assessment of the lower urinary tract. As mentioned previously, the bladder normally fills at low pressures and transitions through phases of filling and sensations. Patients who have OAB may demonstrate detrusor contraction suddenly, which will be identified during urodynamics because Pdet will have a sudden rise and patients will subjectively report urgency. This contraction is termed detrusor instability. Uroflowmetry and voiding pressures are obtained and in OAB will likely reveal no significant abnormalities.

Case Report

A 56-year-old postmenopausal woman presents to the clinic with a 6-month progressive history of urinary frequency, urgency, nocturia, and now incontinent episodes. She states that the symptoms started mildly, but have progressed to the point that she is unwilling to accept the changes she is experiencing. She states she is wearing pads continually and urge incontinence occurs one to four times per day. She states she is much stressed at home and work. She denies dysuria and hematuria. She takes no other medication and has no comorbid conditions. She had a complete hysterectomy at 38 years old. Vaginal examination reveals a slightly atropic vagina though there is no evidence of pelvic organ prolapse. Otherwise, her history and physical are unremarkable. Her 3-day bladder diary reveals oral intake of mostly water throughout the day. On average she has two to three urge incontinent episodes per day. No specific trigger is identified from the diary.

An urodynamic evaluation is performed to evaluate the mechanism of the incontinence. Findings from the urodynamic study include

- Uroflowmetry: Overall it was within normal limits with a Qmax equal to 20 mL/s.
- Postvoidal residual: PVR equals 15 mL.
- Cystometry: Patient had first desire at 50 mL of filling. Pdet rose from 12 cm/H2O to 25 cm/H2O. Patient experienced small amount of leakage. Instillation was discontinued. Pves and Pdet returned to baseline. Filling was reinitiated. At 120 mL of filling the patient again had a Pves and Pdet increase to 25 cm/H2O and subsequent leakage. The patient continued this trend throughout the filling phase and was instructed to void to completion upon an occurrence of an unstable detrusor contraction at 230 mL.
- Leak point pressure: At 150 mL of filling, the patient was instructed to perform the valsalva maneuver. No leakage was noted.
- Pressure flow study: Once patient reported urgency at 230 mL she was instructed to void. No abnormalities were identified. Detrusor pressure during voiding was found to be within normal limits.

Based on the urodynamic study, along with the patient's history and physical, this patient has the diagnosis of OAB. Treatment options for OAB include antimuscarinic/anticholinergic drugs. This classification of pharmacologic agents block muscarinic receptors.[21] The detrusor muscle is stimulated by ACh released from the parasympathetic nervous system. In turn, when the muscarinic receptor is blocked the bladder has a decreased ability to contract, hence decreasing the symptoms of OAB. Other treatment options for this patient would include bladder training and pelvic floor muscle training to inhibit sudden urges. The patient should also begin a form of stress reduction, as stress has been linked to an increased incidence of OAB.[17] The patient will follow up for evaluation of the outcomes of the proposed therapy. If the patient does not have success with the above regimen, more invasive treatment options including botulinum-A toxin (Botox) injected into the bladder and implanted sacral nerve stimulation are available.

SPINA BIFIDA AND NEUROGENIC BLADDER

Myelomeningocele spina bifida is one of the most common causes of neurogenic bladder in pediatric patients. Pathophysiology of neurogenic bladder includes a decreased nerve supply to the bladder that affects the sphincter and detrusor tone.[22] In a child who has normal detrusor function, as the bladder fills, the parasympathetic nervous system is stimulated to contract the detrusor muscle which then allows the bladder to expel urine to the urethra. In a child who has myelomeningocele, negative effects include involuntary contractions of the detrusor that lead to increased incontinence of urine. Complications of untreated neurogenic bladder include renal impairment, upper urinary tract deterioration, UTI, and skin infections caused by incontinence. In fact, approximately 10% to 30% of all children born with myelomeningocele have an abnormal upper urinary tract.[23]

Goals for long-term prognosis are achievement of urinary continence and minimization of any renal deterioration. The focus of treatment of neurogenic bladder relies primarily on alteration of abnormal bladder and detrusor behaviors, specifically suppression of detrusor overactivity. This suppression is achieved, in most cases, through a combination of self catheterization and pharmacologic therapy. Pharmacologic therapy includes the use of anticholinergic/antimuscarinic therapy, specifically oxybutynin (Ditropan), which reduces the spasms of the detrusor muscle allowing for longer intervals between voids, increased voiding volume, and dryness.[24] Most children are also placed on prophylactic antibiotic therapy, mostly trimethoprim (Bactrim), to prevent breakthrough infections.[25] For children who have failed control despite behavioral and pharmacologic therapies, surgical intervention may be warranted.

Case Report

An 8-year-old boy presents to the clinic with complaints of constant dribbling of urine between intermittent catheterizations. Past medical history includes myelomeningocele diagnosed at birth with varying levels of paralysis to both legs. The child's mother reports using clean intermittent catheterization every 3 hours. The mother states the child has previously been dry and has recently experienced increased incontinence between catheterizations. Current medications include oxybutynin (Ditropan) and trimethoprim. The patient denies any pain, fever/chills, hematuria, or changes in the color or odor of the urine output. Urinalysis is negative for presence of bacteria, nitrites, and white blood cells.

An urodynamic evaluation is performed to evaluate bladder dysfunction. Findings from the Urodynamic study include

- Uroflowmetry: It was unable to obtain because of incontinent voiding and inability to initiate void upon command.
- Postvoidal residual: After an incontinent episode, the residual was 50 mL.
- Cystometry: When the bladder reached capacity, the end-filling pressure was 40cm/H_2O. This is the most significant finding for this patient as findings that indicate risk factors for deterioration include a maximum detrusor pressure greater than 40cm/H_2O during filling.[26]
- Leak point pressure: 150 mL were instilled and end-fill pressure reached 40cm/H_2O. At that time, the study was discontinued and the bladder was emptied by way of catheterization.

Urodynamics and Neurogenic Bladder

For children who have spina bifida, yearly urodynamic evaluation through at least 5 years of age is recommended because of the rapid growth during these years.[27] There appears to be no recommendation for serial urodynamic studies as the child continues to age and growth patterns slow. In the case report above, the patient presented with increased incontinence despite pharmacologic therapy and self catheterizations. Urodynamic testing is certainly indicated in cases such as this, when children have continued bladder issues related to failed behavioral and pharmacologic therapy.[24] In this patient's particular case, the end filling cystometry pressure was 40 cm/H_2O. His previous year urodynamic finding indicated a pressure of 25cm/H_2O, which indicates a decrease in bladder compliance, therefore placing the child at risk for upper urinary tract impairment and subsequent renal impairment. Most disturbing for the patient's daily self care is his complaint of dribbling and wetness between catheterizations. Unfortunately, when bladder compliance becomes insufficient, as evidence of this patient's end-filling pressure of 40cm/H_2O, the child also has an increased risk for chronic urinary leakage.[22]

The goal of care for this patient is to achieve and maintain a lower bladder pressure. Becasue medical therapy combined with behavioral therapy has resulted in insufficient bladder compliance, this child is a candidate for more aggressive therapy that may include injections of botulinum-A toxin and surgical therapies. Long-term results are not clear with botulinum-A toxin therapy, however, it seems that this therapy is having efficacy in pediatric patients with neurogenic bladder.[24] Risks for pediatric patients specifically include a lack of evidence on long-term effects of this injection therapy.[25] Surgical correction, which is a last resort, involves an invasive approach to bladder augmentation or urinary diversion. Depending on the specific findings, multiple surgical approaches may be used.

OBSTRUCTIVE VOIDING RELATED TO BENIGN PROSTATIC HYPERPLASIA

Urodynamics has been discussed for its usage in the assessment and diagnosis of urinary incontinence; however, it is also useful in the assessment and diagnosis of obstructive voiding symptoms secondary to BPH. BPH occurs when hyperplasia of the prostate occurs under the influence of hormones in aging men. Because the prostate straddles the urethra, the hyperplasia of the gland can cause obstruction of the flow of urine. Men who have BPH will present with complaints of frequency (caused by incomplete bladder emptying), hesitancy, nocturia, post-void dribbling, and intermittency of urinary stream. These complaints are often treated empirically based on history and physical examination; however, uroflowmetry and other components of urodynamics can contribute objective findings to make the diagnosis.

Uroflowmetry in patients who have BPH will reveal a decreased Qmax and a prolonged voiding time. Additionally, patients will likely have an increased PVR (>100ml). These two components alone can provide needed information to initiate treatment. For complicated cases the other components of urodynamics may provide additional information.

SUMMARY

Voiding dysfunction has profound physical, emotional, and financial ramifications for patients and health care practitioners from all fields. The improvement of diagnostic testing in the area of voiding dysfunction, throughout decades, has resulted in improved outcomes for patients. The components of urodynamic studies can allow practitioners an objective measurement to assist in making a correct diagnosis, hence appropriate interventions. An urodynamic study decreases the risk of a patient undergoing unnecessary surgical procedures. Urodynamics is an invasive procedure, though with the maintenance of sterile technique and patient education it is generally well tolerated with few adverse effects.

REFERENCES

1. Taylor C, Lillis C, LeMone P. Fundamentals of nursing. 5th edition. Philadelphia: Lippincott Williams & Wilkins; 2005. p. 1291–2.
2. Blaivas J, Chancellor M. Atlas of urodynamics. Baltimore (MD): Williams & Wilkins; 1996. p. 3.
3. Cole E, Dmochowski R. Office urodynamics. Urol Clin North Am 2005;32:353–70.
4. Dwyer P, Franzcog F, Frcog C, et al. Evaluation and diagnosis of the overactive bladder. Clin Obstet Gynecol 2002;45(1):193–203.

5. Albaugh K. Urinary dysfunction and urodynamics in the elderly. Urol Nurs Urol Clin North Am 2003;23(2):136–40.

6. Latthe P, Foon R, Toozs-Hobson P. Prophylactic antibiotics in urodynamics: a systematic review of effectiveness and safety. Neurourol Urodyn 2008;27: 167–73.

7. Fowler C. Electromyography. In: Blavis J, Chancellor M, editors. Atlas of urodynamics. Baltimore (MD): Williams & Wilkins; 1996. p. 60–76.

8. Kohli N, Karram M. Urodynamic evaluation for female urinary incontinence. Clin Obstet Gynecol 1998;41(3):672–90.

9. Belal M, Abrams P. Noninvasive methods of diagnosing bladder outlet obstruction in men. Part 2: noninvasite urodynamics and combination of measures. J Urol 2006;176:29–35.

10. Abrams P, Chapple C, Khoury S, et al. Evaluation and treatment of lower urinary tract symptoms in older men. J Urol 2009;181:1779–87.

11. Tanagho E, McAninch J. Smith's general urology. 15th edition. New York: McGraw-Hill; 2000. p. 538–9.

12. Siegel S. Selecting patients for sacral nerve stimulation. Urol Clin North Am 2005; 32:19–26.

13. McGuire E, Cespedes D, Cross C, et al. Videourodynamic studies. Urol Clin North Am 1996;23(2):309–21.

14. Nygaard I, Heit M. Stress urinary incontinence. Obstet Gynecol 2004;104(3): 607–19.

15. Herbruck L. Stress urinary incontinence: an overview of diagnosis and treatment options. Urol Nurs 2008;28(3):186–98.

16. Lewis S, Heitkemper M, Dirksen S, et al. Medical-surgical nursing. 7th edition. St. Louis (MO): Mosby Inc; 2007. p. 1181.

17. Milne J. Behavioral therapies for overactive bladder: making sense of the evidence. J Wound Ostomy Continence Nurs 2008;35(1):93–101.

18. Tyagi S, Thomas C, Hayashi Y, et al. The overactive bladder: epidemiology and morbidity. Urol Clin North Am 2006;33:433–8.

19. Tubaro A, Palleschi G. Overactive bladder: epidemiology and social impact. Curr Opin Obstet Gynecol 2005;17:507–11.

20. ICS factsheet 2 overactive bladder. International Continence Society. Available at: http://www.icsoffice.org. Accessed April 16, 2009.

21. Andersson K, Chapple C, Cardozo L, et al. Pharmacological treatment of overactive bladder: report from the International Consultation on Incontinence. Curr Opin Urol 2009;19:1–15.

22. Wong D, Hockenberry M. Nursing care of infants and children. St. Louis (MO): Mosby Inc; 2003. p. 428–30.

23. Perez L, Wilbanks J, Joseph D, et al. Urological outcome of patients with cervical and upper thoracic myelomeningocele. J Urol 2000;164:962–4.

24. Ellsworth P, Caldamone A. Pediatric voiding dysfunction: current evaluation and management. Urol Nurs 2008;28:249–83.

25. de Jong T, Chrzan R, Klijn A, et al. Treatment of neurogenic bladder in spina bifida. Pediatr Nephrol 2008;23(6):889–96.

26. MacLellan D. Management of pediatric neurogenic bladder. Curr Opin Urol 2009; 19:1–5.

27. Holzbeierlein J, Pope J, Adams M, et al. The urodynamic profile of myelodysplasia in childhood with spinal closure during gestation. J Urol 2000;164:1336–9.

Urinalysis: A Review of Methods and Procedures

Xiaohua Wu, MSN, FNP-BC[a,b,*]

KEYWORDS

- Urinalysis • Renal function • Liver function
- Patient care and assessment

The value of urine as a diagnostic aid in the critical care setting cannot be overemphasized. As a noninvasive source of data, urine reveals a wealth of information about the body's biochemical status. Urine is formed through the process of filtration, reabsorption, and secretion in the glomerulus, tubules, and the collecting ducts within the kidney. Each of these activities can be evaluated by appropriately selected laboratory tests.

It is important for critical care nurses to understand the processes that occur in the renal system and to comprehend the depth of information that can be obtained through an analysis of urine. This article provides an overview of common urine tests and provides information for nurses about urine collection methods. The following discussion will help the critical care nurse describe various urine tests procedures, common urine collection methods, nursing interventions, and patient education important to each study.

URINALYSIS

A routine urinalysis is the most common, convenient, and important screening examination, which provides the health professionals with valuable information about the patient's health status, including indication of renal disease, urinary tract disease, liver disease, diabetes mellitus, and general hydration.[1] Urinalysis is a physical, chemical, and microscopic analysis of the urine. Urine color, appearance, odor, and foam are examined. The pH value; specific gravity; protein, glucose, ketone, nitrite, and bilirubin levels; and presence of red blood cells (RBCs), white blood cell (WBCs), and yeast cells are tested. Specific gravity is measured with a urinometer, and a microscopic examination of the urinary sediment is performed to detect RBCs, WBCs, casts, and crystals.

[a] Vanderbilt University School of Nursing, Nashville, TN, USA
[b] Vanderbilt University Kidney Transplant Center, 912 Oxford House, Nashville, TN 37232, USA
* Vanderbilt University Kidney Transplant Center, 912 Oxford House, Nashville, TN 37232.
E-mail address: xiaohua.wu@vanderbilt.edu

Crit Care Nurs Clin N Am 22 (2010) 121–128
doi:10.1016/j.ccell.2009.10.012
0899-5885/10/$ – see front matter © 2010 Elsevier Inc. All rights reserved.
ccnursing.theclinics.com

Urine samples for routine urinalysis are best collected first thing in the morning. Urine that has accumulated in the bladder overnight is more concentrated, thus allowing for detection of substances that may not be present in more dilute random samples. Urine should be examined within 1 hour after it is passed because some urinary components are unstable. If this is not possible, the sample may be refrigerated until it can be examined. Allowing urine to stand at room temperature can cause the glucose level to drop and ketones to dissipate.[1] Similarly, urinary sediment begins deteriorating within 2 hours of collecting the sample.[2] Also, the precipitation of phosphates in an alkaline urine and growth of bacteria with a resulting change to an alkaline pH may take place.[2,3]

Before collecting the urine sample, the ambulant adult patient may be instructed to clean the external genitalia with cotton wool or toilet tissue and tap water before passing urine. This procedure is no longer performed in many areas, however, and the need for it is debated.[4] By using the clean-catch method, after passing a small amount of urine into the toilet, part of the stream can be collected in a clean container. Approximately, 15 to 30 mL of urine needs to be collected for urinalysis results to be accurate.[1,5,6] A nonambulant patient will require help with positioning the specimen container. If the patient is catheterized, the sample can be taken using a 20-mL sterile syringe, a sterile specimen container with screw-top lid, an alcohol swab, and portable sharps bin. The syringe is inserted into the sample port on the catheter tube. The port should be cleaned with an alcohol swab before and after the procedure. If there is no urine in the tubing, the catheter bag tube should be clamped to allow collection of urine. Specimens should never be taken by emptying the catheter bag, as the urine may be stale, and the tap may be contaminated by microorganisms.[4]

Because many drugs and foods may alter the color, odor, or pH value of the sample, a thorough medication and diet history is necessary for evaluating the data obtained. The time of collection and source of the sample must be noted because this information is important in evaluating the results and in distinguishing normal from abnormal results of routine urinalysis.

Assessment after the test include observing the color, clarity, and odor of the sample. Dipstick tests for glucose, ketones, protein, and blood may be performed on separate portions of the sample, if desired.

TESTS OF RENAL FUNCTION

Renal function tests are an important method of evaluating damage or destruction of renal tissue that results in renal dysfunction. A specific kidney function test is available to measure the kidney's filtration, reabsorption, and secretion abilities. The creatinine clearance test reflects glomerular filtration. The urine concentration test indicates the efficiency of tubular reabsorption, whereas the phenolsulfonphthalein (PSP) test measures renal plasma flow and tubular secretion.

Creatinine Clearance Test

Creatinine is produced as the end product of the catabolism of creatine in skeletal muscle[7] and then cleared primarily by glomerular filtration in the kidney. An adult normally excretes 1.2 to 1.7 g of creatinine in 24 hours. Because muscle mass is usually greater in men than in women, the quantity of creatinine excreted is usually greater in men. Creatinine clearance is the most sensitive indicator of glomerular function. Clearance refers to the number of functioning nephrons, the efficiency with which they function, and the amount of blood entering the nephrons. In general, loss of two-thirds of the nephrons will produce a sharp decrease.[3]

A 24-hour urine specimen is usually preferred for the creatinine clearance study. Routine weekly or biweekly 24-hour creatinine clearance is obtained in many intensive care units to assess renal function. Although shorter period, such as 2-, 6-, or 12-hour, urine samples for creatinine clearance may be used to expedite results and initiate earlier treatment decisions, there is no conclusive evidence that this is an accurate measurement of renal function, particularly in critically ill and injured patients.[7,8] When a 24-hour specimen is required, it is desirable to start collecting it in the morning, usually sometime between 5 and 8 AM. The collection begins when the patient completely empties the bladder and discards that specimen. All urine voided thereafter is collected for the next 24 hours. The next day, at the same time the specimen collection was begun, the patient is instructed to void again. This final void is added to the sample, and the collection ends. In the hospital setting, it is helpful if a reminder to collect all urine is posted in or near the patient's bathroom so that neither the patient nor hospital personnel inadvertently discard any portion of the specimen. The patient should be instructed not to place toilet paper in the specimen container. Patients who use a bedpan should be instructed not to void into a bedpan containing feces. When a 24-hour urine collection is obtained via an indwelling catheter, changing the tubing and drainage bag is required before urine collection for accurate results.

A 24-hour urine specimen should be kept on ice or refrigerated throughout the collection period. If the specimen container is placed in a basin filled with ice, the ice supply will need to be renewed frequently to ensure that the specimen is properly chilled. When the collection is completed, the sample should be properly labeled and transported promptly to the laboratory.

Because 24-hour urine collection is a time-consuming procedure prone to errors and difficult to implement in some clinical settings, a thorough instruction needs to be given to the patient. Furthermore, a 24-hour urine collection delays the results for at least 1 day. A blood specimen for serum creatinine could be ordered before the end or at the beginning of the 24-hour urine test period.[2,7] It should be noted that creatinine clearance tends to be influenced by patient's age, gender, body weight, and surface area.[7–10]

Urine Concentration Test

The concentration test measures the ability of the renal tubules to appropriately absorb water and essential salts. If the kidneys are capable of reabsorbing water, they also are assumed to be capable of reabsorbing vital substances from the glomerular filtrate.[11] Failure to concentrate urine usually indicates the presence of renal damage with a reduction in the number of nephrons capable of reabsorbing water from their tubules. Loss of tubular concentrating ability is one of the earliest indicators of renal disease and may occur before blood levels of urea and creatinine rise.[7]

The concentration of urine may be determined by measuring either the specific gravity or the osmolality of the sample. Often, a single early morning urine specimen is sufficient. A series of timed tests conducted over 12 to 24 hours may be necessary if early morning samples indicate inadequate overnight urine concentrating ability. With the Fishberg test, an attempt is made to maximally concentrate urine through fluid restriction. The patient consumes no fluid from the evening meal until breakfast the next morning. Some laboratories require that the evening meal consist of a high-protein, high-sodium diet with no more than 200 mL of fluid. Patients on low-protein or low-sodium diets often fail to excrete urine with an increased specific gravity because of the lack of sufficient urinary solids.[2,8] Patients should be instructed to maintain a diet adequate in protein and fluids for several days before the test. The patient voids at approximately 10 PM or before retiring and discards this urine. The patient must be instructed to empty the bladder completely at 7, 8, and 9 AM. Collect each specimen in its entirety and label with the appropriate time. Each void during the night should be sent to the laboratory as a separate specimen.[2] The patient is instructed to resume normal fluid intake and diet after the test.

PSP Test

A normal kidney quickly removes an intravenous test dose of the PSP dye from the blood and excretes it in the urine. PSP is a dye that binds to albumin in the bloodstream and, therefore, cannot be excreted through the glomerulus. Measuring the amount of dye excreted in serial urine specimens indicates the efficiency of tubular secretion and renal blood flow. PSP is a dye and gives a pinkish color to urine. Within 2 hours of injection, 75% of the dose is excreted if renal blood flow and tubular function are normal.

The patient should be encouraged to drink 4 to 5 glasses of water during the 30 minutes before the test and a glass of water every 20 minutes during the test to ensure an adequate urine flow. This increases the validity of the test results. Also, the patient should be instructed to empty the bladder completely and discard the urine at the start of the test. Before the test, nurses should obtain a detailed history of any allergies, especially those related to shellfish. Positive findings should be reported to the physician. The anaphylaxis trial is made available for the test before the dye is administered.

A serial of 4 urine samples is collected at 15, 30, 60, and 120 minutes after the intravenous PSP injection. The exact time when the PSP dye is administered intravenously is recorded. Each sample should consist of at least 50 mL. Urine specimens are collected and carefully labeled at the exact times. The bladder must be completely emptied at each collection time because large amounts of residual urine invalidate the test results. If the patient cannot void at the required time, an indwelling catheter (Foley catheter) may be inserted and the specimen obtained. The catheter needs to be clamped between specimen collections.

After the PSP test, the patient is instructed to resume medications if previously withheld. The dye injection site is monitored for inflammation and hematoma formation. The Foley catheter is removed, if inserted for the test, and the patient's voiding pattern is assessed.

Electrolytes (Sodium, Chloride, Potassium, Calcium, Phosphorus, Magnesium)

One of the major functions of the kidney is the regulation of electrolyte balance. Along with the kidneys, the lungs and the endocrine system are also responsible for regulating the distribution of body fluids and the proper balance among electrolytes. Normally, 80% to 90% of the ingested sodium, potassium, and chloride are excreted by the kidneys in the urine. Tests for electrolytes in urine usually involve 24-hour urine collections.

Most of the sodium filtered through the glomerulus is reabsorbed in the proximal renal tubule. Serum and urine sodium concentrations are used to detect changes in water and sodium balance. However, urine sodium determinations are a much more sensitive guide to fluctuations in sodium balance because serum values are of little help in detecting early or subtle electrolyte changes.[12] Increased loss of sodium into the urine is associated with excessive salt intake, diuretic therapy, diabetic ketoacidosis, adrenocortical hypofunction, toxemia of pregnancy, hypokalemia, and excessive licorice ingestion.[13–15] In acute renal disease involving the renal tubules, there may be excessive loss of sodium into the urine, as the tubules are too impaired to reabsorb sodium normally.

Chloride is absorbed into the bloodstream from dietary sodium chloride and is a vital factor in preserving electrical neutrality. Its main function is to counterbalance sodium and act as a buffer during oxygen and carbon dioxide exchange in red blood cells. The kidneys may secrete either chloride or bicarbonate, depending on the acid-base balance of the body.

Urine chloride measurements require a 24-hour urine specimen collected without preservatives and sent to the laboratory in its entirety so that the total volume can be measured. Urine specimens must be collected in clean, dry containers that are free of saline or chloride-containing solutions.

Potassium is filtered through the glomerulus and reabsorbed through the tubules. Potassium plays a major role in influencing the body's water balance, controlling acid-base equilibrium, and regulating the electrical potential in all muscle cells.

Calcium is the most abundant cation in the body, with bone being its major reservoir. Only a small amount of calcium circulates in the blood, which is absorbed into the bloodstream from the small intestine after dietary intake. Total calcium concentration is regulated by the parathyroid hormone, which releases calcium and phosphorus from bone and increases calcium absorption from the intestine. Urine calcium reflects the dietary intake of calcium, the serum calcium level, and the effects of disease entities.

A 24-hour urine specimen is required for urine calcium measurements. Ten milliliters of concentrated hydrochloric acid or glacial acetic acid is added in the 24-hour urine specimen container.[2] Urine specimens for calcium measurement remain stable for 7 days at room temperature.[2,5] High or low calcium content in the diet may affect test results, so patients' dietary intake of milk, cheese, butter, and certain meats and vegetables needs to be assessed. Also, thiazide diuretics can decrease urine calcium level, and drugs containing sodium and magnesium can elevate urine calcium level.

As with calcium, serum contains a relatively small amount of phosphorus, with bone serving as the major reservoir. Phosphorus metabolism is associated directly with calcium metabolism and is regulated by the parathyroid glands and vitamin D. Thus, tests for calcium and phosphorus are usually ordered simultaneously because each value is important to the proper evaluation and interpretation of the other.

Magnesium is a vital coenzyme in the metabolism of carbohydrates, lipids, and proteins and is essential to the maintenance of the macromolecular structure of DNA and RNA. Magnesium also participates in the control of serum electrolyte levels and increases intestinal absorption of calcium. Signs and symptoms of magnesium imbalance are manifested primarily in the central nervous and neuromuscular systems. Urinary measures of magnesium may be used instead of serum measures because changes in magnesium levels are reflected more quickly in the urine than in the blood.

Proteins and Uric Acid

Normally, the urine contains only a scant amount of protein. Excessive amounts of protein in the urine are generally associated with renal disease resulting from glomerular damage and/or impaired renal tubular reabsorption. Part of the screening process in a routine urinalysis is to test the sample for protein. If increased amounts are found, a quantitative 24-hour urine collection is performed.[13–15]

Protein metabolites such as creatinine and uric acid also may be measured in urine. Uric acid is an end product of purine metabolism. Purines are synthesized in the body from the breakdown of cellular nucleic acids or are absorbed by the intestines from the complex nucleoproteins in foods. Dietary sources of purines include organ meats, legumes, mushrooms, spinach, coffee, tea, cocoa, and yeasts. The amount of uric acid produced in the body and the efficiency of renal excretion affect the amount of uric acid found in urine.

Determination of urine uric acid values requires a 50-mL aliquot of a 24-hour urine specimen that has been kept refrigerated throughout the collection period. When uric acid determinations cannot be performed immediately, urine specimens may be refrigerated, as the specimen remains stable for 1 week when refrigerated. Falsely elevated uric acid values may occur with the consumption of nonglucose sugars and various drugs, including ascorbic acid and methyldopa.

TESTS OF LIVER FUNCTION
Pigments (Porphyrins)

Those porphyrins for which urine may be tested include aminolevulinic acid (ALA), porphobilinogen, uroporphyrin, and coproporphyrin. Porphyrins are used in the synthesis of hemoglobin and of any hemoproteins, which are carriers of oxygen. Normal excretion of coproporphyrins is minimal, but the amount excreted rises during liver damage.[16]

The presence of ALA in the urine is associated with lead poisoning which is also found in liver disease (eg, hepatic carcinoma and hepatitis) and in acute intermittent.[17]

Tests for porphyrins usually involve collection of 24-hour urine samples to determine the quantity of the specific substance present. Urine needs to be collected in a dark container containing the preservative sodium carbonate. If a large, clear container is used, protect it from light and refrigerate it.

HORMONES AND THEIR METABOLITES
Cortisol

Cortisol is the predominant glucocorticoid. It is produced and secreted in response to adrenocorticotropin hormone (ACTH), which is from the pituitary gland. ACTH stimulates cortisol production in response to a normal circadian rhythm and suppresses production through a negative feedback inhibition. The rate of cortisol secretion also is affected by physical and psychological stress and low blood glucose levels.[18]

The purpose of urinary measures of cortisol is to detect elevated levels of free cortisol, which may not be apparent in random blood samples. It is one of the best screening tests for confirming the diagnosis of Cushing disease because there is very little overlap between normal and abnormal values.

A 24-hour urine sample is required for cortisol testing. Patients should be instructed to avoid excessive exercise and stress 12 hours before the test. The urine sample should be refrigerated or placed on ice throughout the collection period.

Aldosterone

Aldosterone, a potent mineralocorticoid produced by the adrenal cortex, regulates the transport of electrolyte ions across renal tubular membranes, controlling blood volume and maintaining blood pressure through the retention of extracellular fluid. Aldosterone secretion is stimulated by the renin-angiotensin system to adjust the extracellular fluid volume through the retention of sodium and chloride and the excretion of potassium.[19]

Aldosterone levels are influenced by posture and the state of salt balance, which often may cause normal and abnormal values to overlap. For example, patients who remain upright for 4 hours have aldosterone levels that are approximately 50% of those who remain supine. In addition, a low salt intake and potassium administration generally double aldosterone secretion, whereas sodium administration and potassium deficiency reduce aldosterone secretion. Thus, it is important for the patient to have a normal sodium diet immediately before and during the test.[20]

Urinary aldosterone determinations require a 100-mL aliquot of a 24-hour urine specimen collected in a bottle containing 10 g of boric acid and refrigerated during the collection period. Urine specimens for aldosterone analysis remain stable for 7 days at room temperature. The total 24-hour urine volume should be recorded on the laboratory request slip and the urine collection container.

Human Chorionic Gonadotropin

Human chorionic gonadotropin (hCG) is produced only by the developing placenta after the implantation of the fertilized ovum into the uterine wall, and its presence in urine has been used for decades to detect pregnancy. The first substance associated with pregnancy is hCG, and it is detectable before the onset of clinical symptoms of pregnancy. The primary function of hCG is to maintain the corpus luteum during the first trimester of pregnancy to ensure the adequate production of estrogen and progesterone until the placenta can provide these hormones. Increased concentrations of hCG may be detected in the urine 6 to 8 days after conception, increase dramatically throughout the first trimester of pregnancy, and reach peak concentrations at 8 to 12 weeks of gestation.[21]

Laboratory determinations of hCG are generally used to detect pregnancy within 10 to 14 days of conception; it may also be used to diagnose and monitor several other conditions. Elevated hCG levels may aid in the diagnosis and management of malignant neoplasms because hCG often appears in patients with hydatidiform moles and certain testicular and ovarian germ-cell tumors. Measurement of urinary hCG may be performed on any morning urine specimen with a specific gravity greater than 1.010.

SUMMARY

Urinalysis provides various test values ranging from apparent color, appearance, odor, and foam to diverse physical, chemical, and biologic substance amounts. There is no doubt that much more information can be obtained from urinalysis that is not described in this article. All of this information play a vital role for health professionals to better assess the patient's status and provide thorough health care as needed.

REFERENCES

1. Kee JL. Laboratory and diagnostic tests with nursing implications. 4th edition. Norwalk (CT): Appleton & Lange; 1995.
2. Byrne CJ. Laboratory tests: implications for nursing care. 2nd edition. Menlo Park (CA): Addison-Wesley Publishing Co. Health Sciences Division; 1986.
3. Watson J, Jaffe MS, Cella JH. Nurse's manual of laboratory and diagnostic tests. 2nd edition. Philadelphia: Davis; 1995.
4. Whitfield HN. ABC of urology: Urological evaluation. Br Med J 2006;333:432–5.
5. Simerville JA, Maxted WC, Pahira JJ. Urinalysis: a comprehensive review. Am Fam Physician 2005;71:1153–62.
6. Lifshitz E, Kramer L. Outpatient urine culture: does collection technique matter? Arch Intern Med 2000;160:2537–40.
7. Cherry RA, Eachempati SR, Hydo L, et al. Accuracy of short-duration creatinine clearance determinations in predicting 24-hour creatinine clearance in critically ill and injured patients. J Trauma 2002;53:267–71.
8. Markantonis SL, Agathokleous-Kioupaki E. Can two-, four- or eight-hour urine collections after voluntary voiding be used instead of twenty-four-hour collections

for the estimation of creatinine clearance in healthy subjects? Pharm World Sci 1998;20:258–63.

9. Semeniuk H, Church D. Evaluation of the leukocyte esterase and nitrite urine dipstick screening tests for detection of bacteriuria in women with suspected uncomplicated urinary tract infections. J Clin Microbiol 1999;37:3051–2.

10. Fowlis GA, Waters J, Williams G. The cost-effectiveness of combined rapid tests (Multistix) in screening for urinary-tract infections. J R Soc Med 1994;87:681–2.

11. Houston M, Atwood L, Marroquin R, et al. Uncomplicated urinary tract infection in women. Diagnostic and therapeutic recommendations. Postgrad Med 1999;105: 181–6.

12. Barry HC, Ebell MH, Hickner J. Evaluation of suspected urinary tract infection in ambulatory women: a cost-utility analysis of office-based strategies. J Fam Pract 1997;44:49–60.

13. Cantor SB, Kattan MW. Determining the area under the ROC curve for a binary diagnostic test. Med Decis Making 2000;20:468–70.

14. Lammers RL, Gibson S, Kovacs D, et al. Comparison of test characteristics of urine dipstick and urinalysis at various test cutoff points. Ann Emerg Med 2001;38:505–12.

15. Kunin CM, White LV, Hua TH. A reassessment of the importance of low-count bacteriuria in young-women with acute urinary symptoms. Ann Intern Med 1993;119:454–60.

16. Froom P, Bieganiec B, Ehrenrich Z, et al. Stability of common analytes in urine refrigerated for 24 h before automated analysis by test strips. Clin Chem 2000; 46:1384–6.

17. Khan MA, Shaw G, Paris AMI. Is microscopic haematuria a urological emergency? BJU Int 2002;90:355–7.

18. Van Nostrand JD, Junkins AD, Bartholdi RK. Poor predictive ability of urinalysis and microscopic examination to detect urinary tract infection. Am J Clin Pathol 2000;113:709–13.

19. Chiasson JL, Aris-Jilwan N, Belanger R, et al. Diagnosis and treatment of diabetic ketoacidosis and the hyperglycemic hyperosmolar state. Can Med Assoc J 2003; 168:859–66.

20. Bonnardeaux A, Somerville P, Kaye M. A study on the reliability of dipstick urinalysis. Clin Nephrol 1994;41:167–72.

21. Lohr JA, Portilla MG, Geuder TG, et al. Making a presumptive diagnosis of urinary-tract infection by using a urinalysis performed in an on-site laboratory. J Pediatr 1993;122:22–5.

Stool Studies: Tried, True, and New

Mary Ann Jessee, MSN, RN

KEYWORDS

- Stool studies • Specimen collection • Specimen handling
- Colorectal cancer • Screening • *Helicobacter pylori*
- *Clostridium difficile*

Bowel elimination and associated pathologies are topics often perceived by patients as embarrassing. For patients, the idea of providing a stool sample may evoke fears of discomfort and loss of privacy and dignity. The associated area, sounds, and smells often associated with gastrointestinal (GI) functions illicit unpleasant emotional and physical responses in patients and caregivers. Critical care nurses, despite a high comfort level with the human body, often view the discussion and handling of GI waste as objectionable. This can result in a minimal desire to seek out knowledge on emerging pathologies, tests, and treatments for the GI system. This may be perceived by patients as a lack of knowledge and respect for their individual diagnoses. These stigmas, along with advances in types of studies, warrant an overview of fecal sampling for diagnostic testing and associated nursing implications.

This discussion offers a review of stool composition and elimination patterns and indications for sampling along with guidelines for specimen collection and handling. Stool collection is often a collaborative process between patient and nurse, necessitating education in relation to stool testing. A review of widely known stool studies, indications for sampling, and recent improvements prefaces identification of newly emerging tests, implications for use, patient preferences, and cultural considerations.

STOOL COMPOSITION AND ELIMINATION

The composition of stool and pattern of elimination vary within the population based on age, diet, fluid status, general GI function, medications, and the presence or absence of pathologic processes. Stool naturally contains bile, mucus, shed epithelial cells, bacteria, and other inorganic salts.[1] The character of stool is evaluated on the basis of color, consistency, frequency, odor, amount, and shape.[2] Assessment centers on recognition of changes in the expected pattern or composition for individual patients. Common changes, such as constipation and diarrhea, if of short duration, may be alleviated with basic nursing or pharmacologic intervention. A persistent

Vanderbilt University School of Nursing, 305 Godchaux Hall, 461 21st Avenue South, Nashville, TN 37240, USA
E-mail address: mary.a.jessee@vanderbilt.edu

Crit Care Nurs Clin N Am 22 (2010) 129–145
doi:10.1016/j.ccell.2009.10.006
0899-5885/10/$ – see front matter © 2010 Elsevier Inc. All rights reserved.

change in bowel elimination pattern or stool consistency may accompany serious fluid and electrolyte imbalances and multiple associated problems. Any change in bowel character or pattern accompanied by other symptoms, such as pain, bloating, blood, fat, or parasites in the stool, requires stool sampling for diagnostic purposes (**Table 1**).

PATIENT EDUCATION

Discussions about bowel elimination patterns and associated symptoms are often difficult and embarrassing for patients and may result in reluctance to seek out prompt treatment or information related to lower GI complaints. In the inpatient environment, collection of stool samples is often a collaborative process between nurse and patient. A straightforward, nonjudgmental approach by a nurse regarding topics often sensitive to patients is essential for effective teaching, adequate patient learning, and achievement of expected outcomes. Nurses are more comfortable with bodily functions than the general population but may fail to identify the emotional response of a patient, such as a perceived loss of privacy. Addressing the primary concerns of patients first promotes a trusting relationship and allows patients to concentrate fully on the subsequent instruction. Nurses must be able to evaluate patients' intellectual capability, motivation, cultural perspective, and desire to learn. To this end, it is imperative that nurses adapt their teaching to the specific needs and learning style of the client.[3] Patients who have a thorough understanding are empowered to participate in their care and, as a result, are more likely to experience the motivation needed to follow through with the plan of care.

When educating patients on stool sampling, nurses should include information about the specific test to be conducted, the rationale for that test, the specific procedure for specimen collection, possible results, and a time frame for those results. Patients assisting with or collecting their own sample should be given more detailed instruction on aseptic technique, collection procedure, and maintenance of sample integrity (**Table 2**).

SPECIMEN COLLECTION AND HANDLING

Correct collection procedure and specimen handling are essential to the accuracy of test results. As with all blood and body fluids, stool is a potential contaminate. Collection procedure, volume of sample required, and postcollection specimen handling vary with test type. The amount of stool needed may involve small samples or multiple days of collection depending on the specific test performed. Most tests require that a sample be taken from an expelled fecal mass; however, rectal swabs are sometimes a viable option. Specimen integrity is often affected by temperature variations resulting in the need for special handling dependent on organism and type of test (**Table 3**).

INDICATIONS FOR STOOL SAMPLING

Symptoms and pathologic processes that necessitate stool sampling are many and diverse. Often, there are various types of laboratory and diagnostic testing appropriate for evaluating a patient complaint or GI-type symptoms. Stool testing is initially more preferable compared with use of more costly, time-consuming, or invasive laboratory testing or diagnostic studies. At any point in the lifespan, symptoms, such as prolonged diarrhea, GI pain, abdominal bloating, and changes in stool constituents, including the presence of blood, fat, or parasites, or processes, such as electrolyte imbalances, malabsorption, and maldigestion, may be evaluated by testing of a stool.

Table 1
Abnormal stool characteristics and interventions

Stool Characteristic	Possible Etiology	Nursing Interventions	Possible Stool Test Indicated
Hard, dry, difficult to pass	Inactivity, decreased fluid intake, low-fiber or high-fat diet, medication side effects	Promote peristalsis with ambulation or other activity. Increase fluid intake. Include more sources of fiber in diet. Evaluate medications and intervene to decrease associated side effects.	None
Loose or watery	Liquid diet, food intolerances, viral or bacterial illness, medication side effects	Eliminate associated foods. Introduce bulk-forming foods. Evaluate medications and intervene to decrease associated side effects. Request antidiarrheal medication or bulk-forming supplement.	Culture
Fat	Malabsorption, maldigestion, ingestion or use of oily substances, such as mineral oil, Olestra (oil used in some potato chips), suppositories	Evaluate dietary fat intake: if high, decrease fat intake. Evaluate medications, intervene to decrease associated side effects.	Fecal fat PE-1
Mucus	Excessive straining, inflammation	Investigate etiology of straining, intervene accordingly. Assess for symptoms of heightened inflammatory response, intervene accordingly.	Culture
Blood	GI bleeding, infection, inflammation or irritation	Assess for associated GI symptoms, promptly notify provider, and implement ordered diagnostic testing.	Stool for occult blood, Apt culture
Parasites	Ingestion of infested food or water, other environmental exposure	Notify provider, collect stool sample for organism identification.	Culture
Bloating or pain	Obstruction, infection, intestinal perforation	Assess for associated GI symptoms, notify provider, administer ordered medication, or implement ordered diagnostic testing.	Culture stool for occult blood

Table 2
Guidelines for specimen collection and handling

Specimen Collection and Handling Guidelines	Methods
Prevent spread of pathogens	Observe standard precautions at all times. Instruct patient not to touch sample. Instruct patient to wash hands thoroughly after sample collection.
Maintain sample integrity	Use strict aseptic technique. Instruct patient to defecate into a clean bedpan or container under toilet seat or collect from incontinence pad. Place sample in a designated container and seal. Store samples as recommended until transport to laboratory.
Ensure adequate sample for testing	Know recommended sample size prior to collection. Use recommended collection technique. If using a rectal swab: the swab should be inserted at least 1 in into the rectum and rotated for at least 30 s.
Ensure correct patient identification	Label sample as directed. Complete all necessary laboratory requisitions as directed.
Ensure timely return of test results	Transport to laboratory immediately after collection. If transport is delayed or collection lasts multiple days, store sample as recommended.
Decrease anxiety in the patient	Fully inform patient of procedure, purpose, and results time frame.

Stool sampling is frequently used as a screening tool for the detection of pathologic processes, such as colorectal cancer, through detection of occult blood and may also serve as a means for measurement of organ dysfunction. The noninvasive nature of stool sampling deems it a viable option to improve patients' desire to engage in recommended screening regimens. Stool sampling for identification of pathogens is often used to diagnose infection, predict risk for disease processes, and dictate measures to prevent outbreaks of nosocomial infection.

APT TEST

The Apt test, also referred to as the qualitative fetal hemoglobin stool test, stool for swallowed blood, or Downey test, is used to differentiate between swallowed maternal blood or actual GI bleeding in a newborn.[1] This test should be performed in cases where there is visualized or suspected blood in the meconium of a newborn.[4] Hemoglobin A (present in adult hemoglobin) and hemoglobin F (present in fetal and newborn hemoglobin) react differently to the process of alkaline denaturation. The traditional Apt test uses the differences in process and is performed by adding sodium hydroxide to the stool sample.[4] If maternal blood is present, it fades to a yellow or brownish color.[1,4] The hemoglobin F present in newborn blood is resistant to hydroxide and, therefore, remains red after exposure to the sodium hydroxide.[4]

Table 3
Stool test collection and handling summary

Test	Collection Procedure and Sample Size	Handling Specifications	Results Time Frame
Apt	Small sample	Emergent test: deliver to laboratory for immediate testing.	Immediately visualized
gFOBT	Smear three consecutive samples 3-day diet free of dietary sources of perioxidase; guiac-impregnated card, wooden applicator, developer; Follow manufacturer instructions or testing procedure	Bedside point-of-care test. Perform test within 48 hours of collection.	30 seconds–2 minutes
iFOBT (FIT)	Smear one to two consecutive samples; test card, brush applicator; follow manufacturer instructions for testing procedure.	Must be sent to laboratory for interpretation.	Up to 48 hours
Fecal fat	72-Hour stool collection; precollection diet of 50–150 g fat/day; collect on 4th, 5th, and 6th days of specified diet	Clean containers. Refrigerate specimens during collection. Record date/time of each specimen. Freeze on dry ice for transport to laboratory if test is not performed within 24 hours.	Several days
PE-1	0.1 g stool; one random specimen	Clean container.	Several days
Culture	1-in diameter, 5-mL liquid, or rectal swab if necessary; collect from clean bedpan or container with sterile tongue blade, place in sterile container	Use sterile container. Refrigerate if not sent to laboratory immediately.	48–72 hours
Fecal leukocytes	Small sample	Clean container	48 hours
CTA	Fresh specimen; 25 g solid, 25–50 mL liquid; up to three sequential samples	Use sterile container, no preservative. Deliver to laboratory within 3–4 hours. Transport in dry ice to outside laboratory. Freeze if not performed within 24 hours.	Up to 48 hours
sDNA	Entire bowel movement, 30 g minimum	Freeze and transport on dry ice.	2–3 weeks

Expected results of the Apt include no newborn blood but may include the presence of maternal blood. This test can be performed with as little as a stool stain on a diaper and may also be performed on amniotic fluid and emesis.[1] The major disadvantage of this test is that results are evaluated only by subjective visual interpretation, which may result in inaccurate results.[4] Visualization of results takes only minutes and results are returned swiftly due to the possible emergent nature of associated etiologies.[4] Infrequent use and complicated laboratory processes contribute to the limited availability of the Apt test.[4] As a result, this may cause an unnecessary use of radiographic studies to rule out GI bleeding versus swallowed maternal blood in the newborn.

A new test using a high-performance liquid chromatography (HPLC) method to differentiate between hemoglobin A and hemoglobin F has been shown more sensitive and more specific than the traditional Apt test. The high-performance liquid chromatography method uses cation chromatography to quantify the type of hemoglobin, thus eliminating the need for visual interpretation.[4] This type of test requires equipment usually present in laboratories and has wider availability than the traditional Apt test, which might result in a decrease in the overuse of radiologic studies.[4]

STOOL FOR OCCULT BLOOD

Evaluation of stool for occult blood is the detection of invisible blood in the stool. Indications for this test include routine screening for colorectal cancers, evaluation of GI pain of unknown etiology, and confirmation of bleeding in patients with GI pathologies, including peptic ulcers, esophageal varices, colitis, or diverticulitis.[1,5,6] Expected results are negative. A positive result indicates the need for further diagnostic evaluation, which might include a colonoscopy.[7] Tests used for detection of occult blood include guaiac-based FOBTs (gFOBTs), which identify the presence of hemoglobin (regardless of the source), and fecal immunochemical tests (immunochemical FOBTs [iFOBTs] or fecal immunochemical tests [FITs]), which identify only human hemoglobin.

Guaiac-based Fecal Occult Blood Tests

The gFOBT measures the pseudoperoxidase activity in plant perioxidases and the hemoglobin molecule regardless of its source.[7,8] This high-sensitivity test is offset by a low specificity for colorectal bleeding as the stability of the heme molecule in the GI tract allows for detection of bleeding from any source within the GI tract.[8] Patients must adhere to a 72-hour diet free of nonhuman sources of perioxidase, including meat, poultry, fish, and leafy green vegetables, before testing to avoid false-positive results.[1,5–8] Medications that may cause GI bleeding, such as aspirin and anti-inflammatory agents, iron and oxidizing drugs, and potassium preparations, may cause false-positive results and ascorbic acid use may result in false-negative results.[1,5,6]

The intermittent nature of bleeding from most GI pathologies necessitates the collection of a stool smear from three consecutive bowel movements to improve test sensitivity.[7] Samples are collected with wooden applicators, placed on guiac-impregnated cards, treated per manufacturer instructions, and visually interpreted within 2 minutes.[6] Sensitivity and specificity based on brand of test, specific handling of specimen, and interpreter variability contribute to decreased reliability of gFOBT.[7] Despite limitations, the relatively low cost of guiac-based testing for occult blood and availability as a point-of-care test for use at the bedside make it a likely option for inpatient and outpatient screening.

Fecal Immunochemical Tests or Immunochemical Fecal Occult Blood Tests

FITs react only to antibodies present in human globin, the protein portion of the hemo-globin molecule, rather than plant perioxidases or the heme molecule contained in meats ingested in the diet.[7,8] Additionally, digestive enzymes present in the GI tract degrade the globin as it moves through the GI tract, making positive results more specific to colorectal causes.[7] The number of samples recommended for FIT is one or two smears, although this is an ongoing discussion.[7,8] No pretest restrictions are necessary as upper GI bleeding resulting from existing pathologies or medications does not affect test results. Samples are collected from a toilet bowl with a brush by disrupting the constituents of the feces into the surrounding water and placing the water onto a test card.[9] In addition, high specificity and relatively low cost make it a viable option to replace gFOBT.[7,8]

The most recent iFOBTs actually quantify fecal hemoglobin. Studies suggest that higher hemoglobin concentrations are often the result of progressive pathologic processes.[8] This correlation increases the likelihood of differentiation between adenoma and carcinoma.[8] These tests are not diagnostic but allow providers to deter-mine the necessity for further diagnostic testing.[8]

FECAL FAT

The analysis of fecal fat content confirms the presence of steatorrhea or higher than expected fat content in the stool. A fecal fat test is indicated when a patient produces larger than expected, foul-smelling, greasy stools. A high fat content in the stool may be an indication of a malabsorption or maldigestion of fat. Pathologic processes that may result in malabsorption of fat include Crohn's disease, celiac disease, Whipple's disease, or cystic fibrosis.[5,6] Maldigestion may be a result of pancreatic or bile duct obstruction from gallstones or tumor, chronic pancreatitis, or surgical removal of a portion of the intestine.[5,6,10]

Fecal fat is measured by the fat retention coefficient (the difference between the in-gested fat and the amount of fat in the stool). The expected value is 95% or higher for children and adults. A lower value confirms steatorrhea.[1,5,6] Recommended prepara-tion for the test includes a diet of 100 g of fat per day for 3 days before testing. Sampling requires a collection of all stools for 24 to 72 hours.[1,5,6] Each specimen should be labeled with date and time and specimens should be frozen on dry ice if not delivered to a laboratory within 24 hours.[6] Use of mineral oil, suppositories, oily lubricants, or substances that increase intestinal motility may cause a high value.[1,5,6] A decreased level may result from the consumption of a high-fiber diet, psyllium-based laxatives, or barium.[5,6] Postcollection patients should be instructed to resume a regular diet and pretest medication or treatment regimens and to expect results to take several days.[6]

PANCREATIC ELASTASE-1

When pancreatic dysfunction is suspected, testing for pancreatic elastase-1 (PE-1), an enzyme produced by the pancreas that is detectable in stool, may prove a better option. Fecal PE-1 has been reported to have higher sensitivity and specificity for diagnosing pancreatic insufficiency than fecal fat analysis and is appropriate for use in adults with suspected pancreatic insufficiency and in children suspected of having cystic fibrosis.[11] PE-1 assays are specific to human PE so are unaffected by commonly used animal-based enzyme therapy regimens.[10]

Reference values are as follows: less than 100 μg PE-1/g stool, severe insufficiency; 100 to 200 μg PE-1/g stool, moderate insufficiency; and greater than 200 μg PE-1/g stool, expected pancreatic function.[10] Although results may take several days, testing for PE-1 requires only a small (0.1-g), random stool sample instead of multiple stools, as does the fecal fat analysis, making PE-1 a more convenient option for patients.[10]

STOOL CULTURE

Stool culture, culture and sensitivity when specifically looking for bacteria, and stool for ova and parasites when looking for fungi and parasites are used to identify the presence of an organism in the GI tract.[1,5,6] Samples are exposed to conditions conducive to pathogen growth followed by testing of pathogens for sensitivity to various anti-infective agents. Culture of stool is indicated when there is suspected infection from bacteria, virus, fungi, or parasites. Indications for sampling include diarrhea, abdominal pain or bloating, flatus, and fever.[1] The normal flora of the GI tract is composed of various bacteria and fungi necessary for adequate function. These commonly present organisms can sometimes overgrow and cause infection as a result of immunosuppression or antibiotic use. Opportunistic bacteria, including Salmonella, Shigella, Campylobacter, Staphylococcus, pathogenic *Escherichia coli*, and Clostridium; fungi, including Aspergillus, and Candida; and parasites, such as Ascaris (hookworm), and Strongyloides (tapeworm) can be ingested and cause infection.[1,5,6]

The expected result of a stool culture is negative for pathogens other than expected concentrations of normal GI flora. Specimen collection should be done under strict aseptic technique and samples placed into sterile containers to prevent contamination and false-positive results.[1,5,6] Recommended sample size is a 1-in diameter solid sample, a small amount of liquid stool, or a rectal swab if necessary.[1,5,6] Samples should be refrigerated if not sent immediately to a laboratory.[6] Stool cultures should be obtained before initiation of anti-infective therapy to preserve the viability of the organism and increase the probability of identification.[5] If antibiotic or antifungal therapy has already begun, note the specific medication on the laboratory requisition.[5] Patients should be informed that this process requires 24 to 48 hours for completion.[1,5,6]

FECAL LEUKOCYTES

Stool sampling to identify the presence of fecal leukocytes is indicated to determine if a pathogen or other process is causing breakdown of the colonic mucosal lining and an associated inflammatory response.[6] The presence of fecal leukocytes indicates that organisms, such as Shiga toxin–producing *E coli*, Salmonella, Shigella, or processes, such as inflammatory bowel disease, are present.[6] Antidiarrheal medications should not be prescribed when fecal leukocytes are present.[6] Viral processes do not usually invade the mucosa and are not accompanied by the presence of fecal leukocytes.[6] The results of fecal leukocyte testing are rapidly obtained.[6] This guides the decision of whether or not to initiate antidiarrheal therapy while awaiting stool culture results.

CLOSTRIDIUM DIFFICILE: A CURRENT CHALLENGE

Over the past 20 years, *Clostridium difficile* has emerged as the major cause of the increasing incidence of nosocomial infectious diarrhea and a leading contributor to increasing morbidity and mortality.[12–14] The emergence of a more toxic strain of *C difficile* has contributed to a marked increase in the number of diagnosed hospital-acquired and community-acquired enterocolitis cases in the United States in the past 10 years.[12,14,15] According to the National Inpatient Survey, the incidence of *C difficile* infection doubled from 1999 to 2005 accounting for 76.8 cases per 10,000 patient discharges.[16] In addition, the 2008 Association for Professionals in Infection Control and Epidemiology survey revealed that the prevalence of *C difficile* infection in health care facilities in the United States is 13.1 per 1000 hospitalized patients.[12] This estimate is a 6.5% to 20% increase over previous estimates.[12] Costs incurred with each case of *C difficile* exceed $4000, bringing the estimated total increased health care costs for patients in this study to more than $32 million.[12,16–18]

Risk for development of *C difficile* infection is increased in susceptible populations. Antibiotic therapy is widely thought a major contributor for *C difficile* infection. Antibiotics known to promote multiplication of *C difficile* include cephalosporins, fluoroquinolones, clindamycin, and ampicillin, although any antibiotic therapy is capable of the same results.[13,14] Persons at risk for developing *C difficile* include patients of increasing age and those with underlying disease processes, such as immunocompromising disorders, other infectious processes, inflammatory bowel pathologies, or surgical procedures.[12,14] Patients with pathologic processes requiring the use of proton pump inhibitors are also at significantly higher risk as a result of the resultant decrease in gastric acid secretion and risk for resultant overgrowth of normal flora.[19]

CLOSTRIDIUM DIFFICILE: HOW IT WORKS

C difficile is a toxin-producing, gram-positive bacteria that can cause significant infection in the intestine. Although *C difficile* is present as part of the normal GI flora, it can become pathogenic under certain conditions. The toxins produced, toxin A (enterotoxin) and toxin B (cytotoxin), attack the intestinal lining and trigger inflammatory processes that result in tissue damage and subsequent diarrhea.[12] In healthy individuals, the *C difficile* present in the intestine does not produce toxins and, therefore, causes no symptoms.[20] Antibiotic therapies or other medications resulting in a decline in or change in the composition of the normal flora, or an immunocompromised state, allow *C difficile* to rapidly multiply and place patients at high risk for development of symptoms.[14]

CLINICAL MANIFESTATIONS AND DIAGNOSIS OF CLOSTRIDIUM DIFFICILE INFECTION

Clinical presentation of patients with *C difficile* varies greatly from the asymptomatic to the symptom laden. Associated manifestations of infectious *C difficile* include fever accompanied by abdominal cramping, bloating, frequent watery, foul-smelling diarrhea, and leukocytosis.[1,5,14] Severe cases may progress to include resultant hypovolemia, progression to fulminant colitis, toxic megacolon, and death.[12,14]

Detecting Clostridium Difficile

There are many methods and various recommendations for detection of *C difficile* enterocolitis, including stool culture, clostridial toxin assay (CTA), enzyme immunoassay (EIA), and panels manufactured to include multiple methods of detection. Each test and current recommendations for testing are addressed.

Clostridial toxin assay

C difficile produces two necrotizing toxins: toxin A, an enterotoxin, and toxin B, a cytotoxin. The toxin assay detects the presence of toxin-producing *C difficile*. This is done by examining the effect of the stool on cultured cells. The cellular changes that occur in the presence of toxins indicate a positive result.[20] CTA requires three fresh sequential stool samples (25 g solid or 25–50 mL liquid).[5,6] Samples must be refrigerated, frozen if the test is not performed within 24 hours, and transported on dry ice to a laboratory within 4 hours.[6] The CTA is indicated in patients with diarrhea accompanied by a 5-day or greater course of antibiotic therapy or an immunocompromised state regardless of antibiotic use.[1] CTA is the most sensitive test for *C difficile* but is costly and results may take up to 48 hours.[14,20]

Enzyme immunoassay for Clostridium difficile

EIA directly detects the presence of toxins produced by the *C difficile* organism. This test is available in forms that identify one toxin or both toxins simultaneously. Although the EIA has the advantage of 24-hour result availability, there is a high false-negative percentage due to the need for a comparatively larger presence of toxin to produce a positive result.[14] The recommendation for conduction of three serial EIA tests when the initial test is positive has been shown to increase accuracy of detection by 10%.[14]

Organism detection assays for Clostridium difficile

Use of anaerobic culture, real-time polymerase chain reaction, and common antigen testing can detect the presence of the organism but are incapable of identifying the difference between toxin- and nontoxin-producing strain.[20] Real-time polymerase chain reaction tests allow for detection and quantification of the organism and, therefore, have higher sensitivity than the EIA and produce rapid results. These factors make it as viable an option as the EIA for the detection of *C difficile*.[14]

All strains of *C difficile* produce the enzyme, glutamate dehydrogenase.[21–23] Common antigen testing for the detection of glutamate dehydrogenase is feasible for screening for colonization due to a relatively high sensitivity and specificity. Because antibodies remain in the system after infection is eradicated, however, a positive glutamate dehydrogenase immunoassay should be followed by testing for toxin with a CTA.[20]

PREVENTION AND CONTROL OF *CLOSTRIDIUM DIFFICILE* IN THE INPATIENT ENVIRONMENT

An estimated 3% of healthy adults and 40% of hospitalized patients have been identified as colonized with *C difficile*.[13] Many patients are asymptomatic carriers, however, and serve as a reservoir resulting in shed of pathogenic organisms into the environment and resultant spread of the infection.[12] The ever-increasing number of infected patients indicates the need for widespread diligent implementation of infection control measures. Control of *C difficile* requires a multifaceted approach that includes environmental control, isolation of infected patients, strict hand hygiene protocols, and control of antibiotic use.[12,14,15]

Environmental Control

Environmental reservoirs from which *C difficile* has been cultured include patient rooms, bathrooms, and equipment and the stethoscopes, thermometers, and blood pressure cuffs used to care for patients.[14] *C difficile* spores can remain on contaminated surfaces from months to years.[14] Environmental surfaces should be thoroughly disinfected with a commercially manufactured hypochlorite-based cleaner or appropriately diluted household chlorine bleach.[15] On moist surfaces, *C difficile* may remain viable for up to 6 hours, indicating the need to thoroughly dry all disinfected surfaces.[14,24]

Contact Isolation Precautions

It is recommended that patients with suspected or diagnosed C *difficile* infection should be immediately placed on contact precautions.[12,14] Infected patients should be placed in a private room or in a room with another C *difficile*–infected patient.[25] In addition to surface contamination, C *difficile* has been shown to contaminate the skin and persist on sites, including groin, chest, abdomen, forearms, and hands.[26] This indicates the need for uncompromised use of gowns and gloves by health care personnel on every entrance to the room of patients with C *difficile* infection to prevent transmission to personnel and other patients. Removal of used gowns and gloves must be completed in patient rooms or associated anterooms to ensure isolation of pathogens. Equipment used to care for patients on contact isolation should be disposable, for single patient use, or dedicated to a patient and adequately disinfected at discharge before use with another patient.[27] Meticulous hand washing is imperative after glove removal as contaminants have been cultured from hands after glove removal.[28]

Hand Hygiene Protocol

The Centers for Disease Control and Prevention recommends hand washing with soap and water as opposed to alcohol-based rubs when caring for C *difficile*–infected patients.[21] The friction associated with soap and water hand washing along with the rinsing action of the water result in more effective removal of organisms from the hands.[22] Alcohol-based rubs do not kill C *difficile* spores and have been implicated as a significant contributor to the increasing incidence of C *difficile* infection.[23,29] Although conflicting opinion exists on the topic of soap and water versus alcohol-based rubs, the majority of evidence shows soap and water to be more effective against the spread of C *difficile*.[21,22,30]

Antibiotic Restriction

Prudent and responsible usage of antibiotic agents known to contribute to C *difficile* infection is an integral piece of the multifaceted approach to limiting outbreaks.[12,27,31] Fluoroquinolones and cephalosporins are widely known as inducers of C *difficile* infection and clindamycin and penicillins.[1,5,6,12–14] Other studies suggest outbreaks can be stalled with enhanced infection control measures alone.[15] Recommended supportive and pharmacologic care includes discontinuation of implicated anti-infective agents, fluid and electrolyte supplementation, avoidance of antiperistaltic medications, and oral vancomycin and metronidazole therapy.[13]

EMERGING STOOL TESTS AND SCREENING RECOMMENDATIONS

As with any discipline, laboratory testing continues to evolve. The development of more efficient, cost-effective, practical methods of testing and screening for certain organisms and pathologies indicates a need for inquiry into emerging tests. Health care consumers are becoming increasingly savvy and are an integral part of the health care team. Patients continue to demand faster, less-invasive, more cost-effective screenings and treatments and are becoming the driving force behind the development of those types of health care products.

Fecal DNA Tests for Cancer Screening

Colorectal cancers are the third leading cause of cancer in men and women.[32] Although there continue to be significant disparities in minority groups, the incidence of colorectal cancer has been decreasing over the past 20 years. This is most likely the result of increased adherence to screening guidelines, resulting in early detection.[32] Ever-increasing patient knowledge, advancement in testing, and rising costs for cancer care are changing the face of cancer prevention and early detection. The recommendations for colorectal screening include testing of stool for DNA variants as a viable alternative to traditional FOBT. Current ACS-MSTF 2008 screening guidelines for colorectal cancer include sDNA testing as an option along with FOBT and FIT for identification of early-stage colorectal cancers.[7]

Progression from adenoma to carcinoma may take as long as a decade. Therefore, the identification and removal of adenomas before development into carcinoma is a primary goal of screening for colorectal cancer.[7] DNA in the cells of neoplastic tissue changes as it goes through carcinogenesis. The sDNA screen detects those genetic mutations in the cells that are shed into the stool from the mucosal lining.[33] Because all tumors do not exhibit the same genetic mutations, sDNA tests are formulated to target multiple mutations.[7]

Comparison of Fecal Occult Blood Testing and DNA for Cancer Screening

Although FOBT (gFOBT and FIT) is valuable for the detection of bleeding from adenomas and cancerous lesions, this bleeding is most often intermittent, decreasing the likelihood of detection. The colonic mucosal lining consistently sheds cells that are easily identifiable in the stool.[33,34] Neoplastic cells shed at a higher rate than normal cells and are detectable at minimal levels.[33] This may result in a significant increase in the early detection of precancerous adenomas.

Advantages of sDNA as a screening for colorectal cancer over FOBT include the stability of DNA during storage and transport, lack of pretesting dietary restrictions, and high DNA stability in the GI tract and stool.[35,36] Although sDNA testing is sensitive to DNA changes, specificity for certain gene changes is low. This increases the likelihood of detection of neoplasia proximal to the colon.[37] Stool sampling for sDNA requires minimum collection of 30 g of the entire bowel movement.[9] Samples must be frozen and transported to a laboratory per test manufacturer instructions and results may take several weeks.[9] A positive sDNA test should be followed by colonoscopy or other radiographic testing to identify the exact location of the lesion.[37]

Detection of Aerodigestive Cancer with Stool Samples

GI cancers proximal to the colon are often diagnosed at a late stage and result in twice the number of deaths per year as colorectal cancers.[37] Aerodigestive cancers, those arising from the lungs, esophagus, gastric mucosa, and pancreas, may shed cells into the GI tract in sputum, saliva, or bile.[33,36,37] As a result of the stability of shed DNA in the GI tract, it is possible to detect these cancers at an early stage.[36] A combined fecal analysis to detect cancer at multiple sites would guide further diagnostic testing and result in overall decreased cost and morbidity.[37] Although minimal studies exist, the emergence of the sDNA test as a promising tool for early identification of neoplasia proximal to the colon warrants further investigation.

Stool Testing for Helicobacter Pylori

Helicobacter pylori infection has been found to be a significant risk factor for the development of peptic ulcer disease, chronic gastritis, and gastric cancer.[38,39] It is speculated that eradication of *H pylori* infection would significantly decrease the incidence of gastric cancer.[39] These findings have driven recent research toward more effective methods for detection of infection and confirmation of eradication after treatment.[39,40]

Conventional diagnosis of *H pylori* infection includes invasive endoscopic biopsy, histology, culture, and noninvasive techniques, such as urea breath testing and now stool testing.[41] Noninvasive stool screening for *H pylori* in clients with GI disease and associated problems is becoming more cost effective and more readily available. As a result, stool antigen tests are beginning to be used to confirm diagnosis and to confirm eradication of *H pylori* after treatment.[42]

Stool antigen testing is emerging as the alternative to the cost-prohibitive urea breath testing.[40] EIAs screen for polyclonal antibodies to *H pylori* and are widely available and have relatively low cost and rapid results return.[41] EIAs have variable sensitivity and specificity, however, and are not capable of confirming eradication after treatment due to the long-term persistence of antibodies to *H pylori*.[41]

Newly developed immunochromatographic tests use monoclonal antibodies to detect *H pylori* antigens and have higher sensitivity for identification of infection and eradication after treatment as opposed to EIA.[42] As a result of recent advancement, the use of stool antigen testing for primary diagnosis and post-therapy eradication confirmation has been approved by the Food and Drug Administration.[42] This nod to the significance of *H pylori* in the development of GI pathologies has implications for improving screening rates, early detection, and resultant prevention of morbidity and mortality.

PATIENT PREFERENCE AND ADHERENCE TO SCREENING RECOMMENDATIONS

Current studies confirm that patients have a desire to be informed participants in decisions being made about their health care, including the choice of screening method for colorectal cancer.[43–45] Patient preferences are influenced by knowledge of test attributes, value placed on those attributes, and level of provider communication and cultural competence.[45,46] Studies show that although many patients who are most concerned about comfort opt for the most technologically advanced, noninvasive tests, other patients concerned about accuracy continue to opt for traditional

---

Box 1
American Cancer Society and US Multi-Society Task Force on Colorectal Cancer screening guidelines

Beginning at age 50, men and women should begin screening with one of the examination schedules below:

Fecal occult blood test (FOBT) or fecal immunochemical test (FIT) every year

Fecal DNA test (stool DNA [sDNA]) every 5 years[a]

Flexible sigmoidoscopy every 5 years

Annual FOBT or FIT and flexible sigmoidoscopy every 5 years[b]

Double-contrast barium enema every 5 years

Colonoscopy every 10 years

Virtual colonoscopy (CT colonoscopy) every 5 years[c]

[a] Recommendations for frequency of sDNA screening are based on current manufacturer suggestions. American Cancer Society–US Multi-Society Task Force on Colorectal Cancer (ACS-MSTF) determined that based on current evidence, the interval for screening is uncertain and needs further research.
[b] Combined testing is preferred over annual FOBT or FIT, or flexible sigmoidoscopy, every 5 years alone. People who are at moderate or high risk for colorectal cancer should talk with a doctor about a different testing schedule.
[c] 5-Year interval appropriate for average-risk adults with negative initial CT colonoscopy.

colonoscopy.[45,46] When fully informed and given the choice, patients most often prefer the most noninvasive and convenient and least complicated screening available.[43,44] Availability of newer, less-invasive tests and provider sensitivity to patient preferences are significant contributors to the goal of increasing adherence to ACS screening guidelines and decreasing colorectal cancer related morbidity and mortality (**Box 1**).[32,46]

Common disparities, including ethnicity and socioeconomic status, may also contribute to a lack of adherence to colorectal screening recommendations and resultant morbidity.[32] Although there is no marked difference in preferences for screening based on race/ethnicity, an identified decreased level of knowledge about screening methods in the African American population dictates the need for improved communication between patients and providers.[45,47] Increasing ethnic diversity and resultant language barriers often deters adequate explanation of test features, thus affecting patient choice.[32,46] Cost of screening is noted by patients as a significant determinant for their choice of whether or not to screen and the choice of which test to use.[47] A higher percentage of African Americans and Latinos compared with whites live in poverty and are uninsured or underinsured, resulting in decreased adherence to screening guidelines and a higher mortality rate from cancer-related deaths.[32]

SUMMARY

Laboratory technology is rapidly advancing in response to pathogen adaptation, growing health care cost, and patient demand for quick, convenient screening methods. The increasing spread of pathogens capable of adverse effects on individuals, the hospital environment, and the community calls for diligent implementation of the most currently recommended measures of control to prevent associated morbidity and mortality. Frequent review of even those topics of lesser interest is paramount in the provision of best nursing practice.

REFERENCES

1. Pagana KD, Pagana TJ. Mosby's manual of diagnostic and laboratory tests. 3rd edition. St. Louis (MO): Mosby; 2006.
2. Potter PA, Perry AG. Bowel elimination. In: Hall A, Stockert PA, editors. Fundamentals of nursing. 7th edition. St. Louis (MO): Mosby; 2009. p. 1174–218.
3. Hess LM. Making community health care culturally correct. Am Nurse 2009;4(5): 13–5.
4. Chen D, Wilhite TR, Smith CH, et al. HPLC detection of fetal blood in meconium: improved sensitivity compared with qualitative methods. Clin Chem 1998;44(11): 2277–80.
5. LeFever-Kee J. Laboratory and diagnostic tests with nursing implications. 8th edition. Upper Saddle River (NJ): Pearson Education; 2010.
6. Chernecky CC, Berger BJ. Laboratory tests and diagnostic procedures. 5th edition. St. Louis (MO): Saunders; 2008.
7. Levin B, Lieberman DA, McFarland B, et al. Screening and surveillance for the early detection of colorectal cancer and adenomatous polyps, 2008: a joint guideline from the American Cancer Society, the US Multi-Society Task Force on Colorectal Cancer, and the American college of radiology. Gastroenterology 2008;134(5):1570–95.
8. Young GP, Cole S. New stool screening tests for colorectal cancer. Digestion 2007;76(1):26–33.

9. Greenwald B. A comparison of three stool tests for colorectal cancer screening. Medsurg Nurs 2005;14(5):292–9.

10. Erickson JA, Aldeen WE, Grenache DG, et al. Evaluation of a fecal pancreatic elastase-1 enzyme-linked immunosorbent assay: assessment versus an established assay and implication in classifying pancreatic function. Clin Chim Acta 2008;397(1–2):87–91.

11. Stein J, Jung M, Sziegoleit A, et al. Immunoreactive elastase 1: clinical evaluation of a new noninvasive test of pancreatic function. Clin Chem 1996;42(2): 222–6.

12. Jarvis WR, Schlosser J, Jarvis AA, et al. National point prevalence of *Clostridium difficile* in US health care facility inpatients, 2008. Am J Infect Control 2009;37(4): 263–70.

13. Bartlett JG. Narrative review: the new epidemic of *Clostridium difficile*-associated enteric disease. Ann Intern Med 2006;145(10):758–64.

14. Hookman P, Barkin JS. *Clostridium difficile* associated infection, diarrhea, and colitis. World J Gastroenterol 2009;15(13):1554–80.

15. Salgado CD, Mauldin PD, Fogle PJ, et al. Analysis of an outbreak of Clostridium difficile infection controlled with enhanced infection control measures. Am J Infect Control 2009;37(6):458–64.

16. Elixhauser A, Jhung M. Clostridium difficile-associated disease in US hospitals, 1993–2005. HCUP statistical brief No. 50, April 2008. US Agency for Healthcare Research and Quality, Rockville, MD. Available at: http://www. hcup-us.ahrq.gov/reports/statbriefs.sb50.pdf. Accessed May 25, 2009.

17. Dubberke ER, Reske KA, Olsen MA, et al. Short and long-term attributable costs of *Clostridium difficile*-associated disease in nonsurgical inpatients. Clin Infect Dis 2008;46(4):497–504.

18. Lawrence SJ, Puzniak LA, Shadel BN, et al. *Clostridium difficile* in intensive care unit: epidemiology, costs, and colonization pressure. Infect Control Hosp Epidemiol 2007;28(2):123–30.

19. Yearsley KA, Gilby LJ, Ramadas AV, et al. Proton pump inhibitor therapy is a risk factor for *Clostridium difficile*-associated diarrhea. Aliment Pharmacol Ther 2006; 24(4):613–9.

20. Reyes RC, John MA, Ayotte DL, et al. Performance of TechLab *C. diff* quik check and Techlab *C. difficile* tox a/b II for the detection of *Clostridium difficile* in stool samples. Diagn Microbiol Infect Dis 2007;59(1):33–7.

21. Boyce JM, Pittet D. Guideline for hand hygiene in health-care settings: recommendations of the healthcare infection control practices advisory committee and the HICPAC/SHEA/APIC/IDSA hand hygiene task force. Infect Control Hosp Epidemiol 2002;23(Suppl 12):S3–20.

22. Siegel JD, Rhinehart E, Jackson M, et al. Healthcare infection control practices advisory committee 2007 guideline for isolation precautions: preventing transmission of infectious agents in healthcare settings, June 2007. Available at: http://www.cdc.gov/ncidod/dhqp/gl_isolation.html. Accessed May 26, 2009.

23. Boyce JM, Ligi C, Kohan C, et al. Lack of association between the increased incidence of *Clostridium difficile*-associated disease and the increasing use of alcohol-based hand rubs. Infect Control Hosp Epidemiol 2006;27(5):479.

24. Mayfield JL, Leet T, Miller J, et al. Environmental control to reduce transmission of *Clostridium difficile*. Clin Infect Dis 2000;31(4):995–1000.

25. Garner JS. Guidelines for isolation precautions. Hospital infection control practices advisory committee. Infect Control Hosp Epidemiol 1996;17(1):53–80.

26. Bobulsky GS, Al-Nassir WN, Riggs MM, et al. *Clostridium difficile* skin contamination in patients with *C. difficile*-associated disease. Clin Infect Dis 2008;46(3): 447–50.

27. Muto CA, Blank MK, Marsh JW, et al. Control of an outbreak of infection with the hypervirulent *Clostridium difficile* BI strain in a university hospital using a comprehensive "bundle" approach. Clin Infect Dis 2007;45(10):1266–73.

28. Doebbeling BN, Pfaller MA, Houston AK, et al. Removal of nosocomial pathogens from the contaminated glove. Implications for glove reuse and handwashing. Ann Intern Med 1988;109(5):394–8.

29. Gordin FM, Schultz ME, Huber RA, et al. Reduction in nosocomial transmission of drug-resistant bacteria after introduction of an alcohol-based handrub. Infect Control Hosp Epidemiol 2005;26(7):650–3, 672.

30. McDonald LC. *Clostridium difficile*: responding to a new threat from an old enemy. Infect Control Hosp Epidemiol 2005;26(8):672–5.

31. Gerding DN, Johnson S, Peterson LR, et al. *Clostridium difficile*-associated diarrhea and colitis. Infect Control Hosp Epidemiol 1995;16(8):459–77.

32. American Cancer Society. Cancer facts & figures 2008. Atlanta (GA): American Cancer Society; 2008.

33. Osborn NK, Ahlquist DA. Stool screening for colorectal cancer: molecular approaches. Gastroenterology 2005;128(1):192–206.

34. Ahlquist DA, Sargent DJ, Loprinzi CL, et al. Stool DNA and occult blood testing for screen detection of colorectal neoplasia. Ann Intern Med 2008; 149(7):441–50.

35. Loganayagam A. Faecal screening of colorectal cancer. Int J Clin Pract 2007; 62(3):454–9.

36. Greenwald B. The stool DNA test: an emerging technology in colorectal cancer screening. Gastroenterol Nurs 2005;28(1):28–32.

37. Ahlquist DA. Next-generation stool DNA testing: expanding the scope. Gastroenterology 2009;136:2068–73.

38. Asaka M, Kimura T, Kato M, et al. Possible role of *Helicobacter pylori* infection in early gastric cancer development. Cancer 1994;73(11):2691–4.

39. Ito M, Takata S, Tatsugami M, et al. Clinical prevention of gastric cancer by *Helicobacter pylori* eradication therapy: a systematic review. J Gastroenterol 2009; 44(5):365–71.

40. Blanco S, Forne M, Lacoma A, et al. Comparison of stool antigen immunoassay methods for detecting *Helicobacter pylori* infection before and after eradication treatment. Diagn Microbiol Infect Dis 2008;61(2):150–5.

41. Chey WD, Wong BC, Practice Parameters Committee of the American College of Gastroenterology. American College of Gastroenterology guideline on the management of *Helicobacter pylori* infection. Am J Gastroenterol 2007;102(8): 1808–25.

42. Gisbert JP, de la Morena F, Abraira V. Accuracy of monoclonal stool antigen test for the diagnosis of *H. pylori* infection: a systematic review and meta-analysis. Am J Gastroenterol 2006;101(8):1921–30.

43. Itzkowitz SH, Jandorf L, Brand R, et al. Improved fecal DNA test for colorectal screening. Clin Gastroenterol Hepatol 2007;5(1):111–7.

44. Schroy PC, Heeren TC. Patient perceptions of stool-based DNA testing for colorectal cancer screening. Am J Prev Med 2005;28(2):208–14.

45. Ling BS, Moskowitz MA, Wachs D, et al. Attitudes toward colorectal cancer screening tests. A survey of patients and physicians. J Gen Intern Med 2001; 16(12):822–30.

46. Hawley ST, Volk RJ, Krishnamurthy P, et al. Preferences for colorectal cancer screening among racially/ethnically diverse primary care patients. Med Care 2008;46(Suppl 9):S10–6.

47. Ruffin MT, Creswell JW, Jimbo M, et al. Factors influencing choices for colorectal cancer screening among previously unscreened African and Caucasian Americans: findings from a triangulation mixed methods investigation. J Community Health 2009;34(2):79–89.

Index

Note: Page numbers of article titles are in **boldface** type.

Crit Care Nurs Clin N Am 22 (2010) 147–160
doi:10.1016/S0899-5885(09)00121-X
0899-5885/10/$ – see front matter © 2010 Elsevier Inc. All rights reserved.

ccnursing.theclinics.com

Moving?

Make sure your subscription moves with you!

To notify us of your new address, find your **Clinics Account Number** (located on your mailing label above your name), and contact customer service at:

Email: journalscustomerservice-usa@elsevier.com

800-654-2452 (subscribers in the U.S. & Canada)
314-447-8871 (subscribers outside of the U.S. & Canada)

Fax number: 314-447-8029

Elsevier Health Sciences Division
Subscription Customer Service
3251 Riverport Lane
Maryland Heights, MO 63043

*To ensure uninterrupted delivery of your subscription, please notify us at least 4 weeks in advance of move.

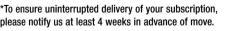